A. Thiede, Y. Hiki, G. Keil

Philipp Franz von Siebold and His Era

Springer

Berlin
Heidelberg
New York
Barcelona
Hong Kong
London
Milan
Paris
Singapore
Tokyo

A. Thiede Y. Hiki G. Keil

Philipp Franz von Siebold and His Era

Prerequisites, Developments, Consequences and Perspectives

With 46 Figures and 4 Tables

15. 2. 2000
Udo Pauli

Springer

Professor Dr. Arnulf Thiede
Direktor der Chirurgischen Universitätsklinik
und Poliklinik Würzburg
Josef-Schneider-Straße 2
97080 Würzburg
Germany

Professor Dr. Gundolf Keil
Institut für Geschichte der Medizin
der Universität Würzburg
Oberer Neubergweg 10a
97074 Würzburg
Germany

Professor Dr. Yoshiki Hiki
Professor emeritus of Kitasato University
1-10-8 Tsuruma
Machida, Tokyo 194-0004
Japan

ISBN 3-540-64185-8 Springer-Verlag Berlin Heidelberg New York

Die deutsche Bilbiothek – CIP Einheitsaufnahme
Phillip Franz von Siebold and his era: prerequisites, developments, consequences and perspectives / A. Thiede... (ed.). – Berlin; Heidelberg; New York; Barcelona; Budapest; Hong Kong; London; Milan; Paris; Singapore; Tokyo: Springer, 2000

Production: PRO EDIT GmbH, D-69126 Heidelberg
SPIN: 10650970 18/3136-5 4 3 2 1 0 Printed on acid-free paper

Contents

List of Contributors

Beireis, Udo
Berufliches Fortbildungszentrum der Bayerischen Wirtschaft
Buchbrunner Straße 53
97318 Kitzingen
Germany

Berchem, Theodor, Professor Dr.
Präsident der Universität Würzburg
Sanderring 2
97070 Würzburg
Germany

Berglehner, Andreas, Dr.
Chirurgische Universitäts-Klinik und Poliklinik Würzburg
Josef-Schneider-Straße 2
97080 Würzburg
Germany

Beukers, Harms, Professor Dr.
Valk Boumannweg 40
2352 JD Leiderdorp
Netherland

Deltz, Eberhardt, Professor Dr.
Friedrich-Ebert-Krankenhaus
Chefarzt der Chirurgischen Abteilung
Friesensstraße 11
24534 Neumünster
Germany

Dettelbacher, Werner
Johannes-Kepler-Straße 20
97074 Würzburg
Germany

Hiki, Sumiko
Essayist
1-10-8 Tsuruma
Machida, Tokyo 194-0004
Japan

Hiki, Yoshiki, Professor Dr.
Professor emeritus of Kitasato University
1-10-8 Tsuruma
Machida, Tokyo 194-0004
Japan

Keil, Gundolf, Professor Dr. Dr.
Institut für Geschichte der Medizin
der Universität Würzburg
Oberer Neubergweg 10a
97074 Würzburg
Germany

Klein-Langner, Wolfgang
Vorsitzender der Siebold-Gesellschaft e.V.
Frankfurter Straße 87
97082 Würzburg
Germany

Kraas, Ernst, Professor Dr.
Krankenhaus Moabit
Chefarzt der I. Chirurgischen Abteilung
Turmstraße 21
10559 Berlin
Germany

Kreiner, Josef, Professor Dr.
Universität Bonn
Japanologisches Seminar
Regina-Pacis-Weg 7
53113 Bonn
Germany

Kutsuzawa, Nobukata, Professor Dr.
Research Insitute of Civilization
Tokai University
1117 Kitakaname
Hiratsuka, Kanagawara, 259-12
Japan

Miyasaka, Masahide, Professor Dr.
Shiroyama-Dai 2-36-10
Nagasaki-Shi
Nagasaki Ken
Japan

Thiede, Arnulf, Professor Dr.
Direktor der Chirurgischen Universitätsklinik
und Poliklinik Würzburg
Josef-Schneider-Straße 2
97080 Würzburg
Germany

Wilms, Klaus, Professor Dr.
Direktor der Medizinischen Poliklinik
der Universität Würzburg
Klinikstraße 8
97070 Würzburg
Germany

CHAPTER 1

Introduction

Th. Berchem

Since its foundation 400 years ago, Würzburg University has followed its purpose of safeguarding tradition and acting as a meeting point for scientists from home and abroad; in short, it is a forum for national and international exchange, in accordance with its memorandum of establishment. The historic role of Würzburg University has been accentuated by its faculty of medicine, surgery in particular. One name, indeed, illuminates its excellent scientific reputation, a name representing a whole dynasty of scholars: Siebold. This year we celebrate the 200th anniversary of Philipp Franz von Siebold's birth. He is one of Würzburg's most famous scholars. However, we should remember that his grandfather, Carl Caspar, originally contributed to a considerable enhancement of this university's reputation: he was the founder and first head of surgery. (I like the idea that he came from my hometown of Nideggen in the Eifel region, but this is only of marginal interest.)

When Carl Caspar came to Würzburg in 1760, the medical faculty consisted of five students. Since then, the total number has grown to 20,000. In 1760 Würzburg University was much different from nowadays. Medicine at Würzburg during the eighteenth century meant the Juliusspital, a very famous hospital at that time and which still exists today. The garden pavilion of that hospital was Germany's first institution for anatomy. It can thus be said that Carl Caspar initiated a renaissance of Würzburg University which was later continued by Döllinger, Schönlein, Heine, Koelliker, Rindfleisch and many other great natural scientists such as Semper, Sachs, Boveri and Röntgen.

There is no doubt that the Siebold family made an important contribution to the good reputation of Würzburg's medical faculty: Carl Caspar was professor of anatomy, surgery and obstetrics. Later, three of his four sons simultaneously accepted chairs in medicine. So the jocular rumour spread, which soon after was repeated with near devotion and respect, about the "Academia Sieboldiana Herbipolensis". The Siebolds' academy, naturally, radiated far beyond Würzburg's walls. This meant that at least 200 years ago surgery became an academic discipline, although it had previously only been regarded as merely practical subject. Medicine finally had become a university discipline due to scientific developments and several successful surgical accomplishments between 1750 and 1850. For Würzburg this is equated with the name of Siebold.

Philipp Franz von Siebold, grandson of Carl Caspar, was born in 1796. Nowadays he is considered the founder and promotor of German–Japanese relations. He followed his family's tradition, studied medicine at Würzburg and attained a doctorate with honours in medicine, surgery and obstetrics. He actuelly never delivered his thesis "De Lingua", but wrote to his uncle: "I will close with the repeated promise that I will honor the name of Siebold and, if Heaven agrees, maintain it in the memory of Würzburg." This promise seems to encapsulate all his various research interests, which often seemed adventurous.

"So öffnet sich den jüngeren Freunden des Orients eine Pforte nach der anderen, um die Geheimnisse jener Urwelt kennenzulernen..." ("So one door after the other opens for the new friends of the Orient to penetrate the mysteries of that primeval world...") are the words of the old master Goethe in his "West-Östlicher Divan". No one has described better than Goethe the charm of travelling, when you absorb other worlds and gain human and scientific knowledge and philosophic sensitivity.

From Würzburg, Siebold went abroad and reached Nagasaki under a Dutch flag. There he intended to establish a relationship with the Land of the Rising Sun in his role as a physician and natural scientist. From his first journey to Japan he brought back so many plants, animals and preparations that a whole group of scholars was occupied for more than 15 years in recording and describing them. He made an essential contribution to the spreading of knowledge about Japan in Germany and the rest of Europe at a time when Japan still preferred its self-imposed isolation. By his various medical, scientific and publishing endeavours, Siebold established important and stable links between Germany and Japan. His fame soon spread, and his home university conferred an honorary doctor's degree on him in 1833.

Siebold's most important contributions, however, consisted of his various advisory activities in politics, as a mediator between different worlds, nations and cultures and as a coordinator of sciences who transcended frontiers. He initiated relationships that still continue today, 200 years later. Siebold in fact discovered Japan for Europe as a scientist, not as a geographer, and with his remarkable personality he was a pioneer in creating a close understanding between the two regions which deserves to be cultivated.

The 73rd Bavarian Surgical Congress in Würzburg, presided over by Prof. Dr. med. Arnulf Thiede in July 1996, was held to commemorate Philipp Franz von Siebold's 200th birthday, underlining the *genius loci herbipolensis.* At Siebold's place of birth and activity, this meeting of prominent surgeons discussed current problems in modern surgery and honoured Siebold's name. I like the idea of combining this surgical congress in Würzburg with Siebold and his birthday, thus commemorating this outstanding physician and explorer. Many people do not yet know that Siebold was a citizen of Würzburg. I wish to thank all the German and Japanese authors for spontaneously agreeing to give us some insight into Siebold's adventurous life. Let us regard their reports as evidence of the reciprocity between Japan and Germany initiated by Siebold and as a way of intensifying this relationship.

There is also an important message we can learn from Siebold's work: his way in which he cultivated tradition and science but, above all, the way in which he initiated peaceful contacts between people. I sincerely wish that there might be further ties between our nations. Würzburg could contribute much with its historical importance and connections, especially in view of the cooperation agreement between the medical faculties of Nagasaki and Würzburg.

CHAPTER 2

Prerequisites for the Reintegration of Surgery into Academic Medicine Before 1850*

A. Thiede, A. Berglehner, G. Keil

Obstacles to the Development of Modern Surgery

If one were to distinguish modern surgery from medieval surgery, modern surgery, as we know it, would be only 150 years old. Medieval surgery was dominated by pain and infection. These were regarded as normal reactions of nature (Rüster 1986).

In January 1845 the dentist Horace Wells tried to demonstrate the first nitrous oxide anesthesia in the operating theater of Massachusetts General Hospital in Boston, USA, which seemed to be a failure. However, he had opened the first chapter of successful modern anesthetic technique. At the same place, William T.G. Morton was more successful with ether anesthesia and, thus, overcame the problem of pain, the most terrifying obstacle in medieval surgery. Until that time, pain had rigorously limited the possibilities for surgical activities. Finally, at least one obstacle in the development of modern surgery had been surmounted when Morton demonstrated the first narcosis during an operation by the surgeon Warren (Fig. 1) in Boston on 16 October 1846 (Ridder 1993).

But what about infection, the second major obstacle hindering surgery in the abdominal cavities?

The gynecologist Ignaz Semmelweis was the first to think of finding a way out of the deadly hell of fever and suppuration. This happened long before the detection of bacteria by Pasteur,

---

* All the illustrations are from the Institute for History of Medicine at the University of Würzburg and have been printed with the kind permission of Prof. G. Keil.

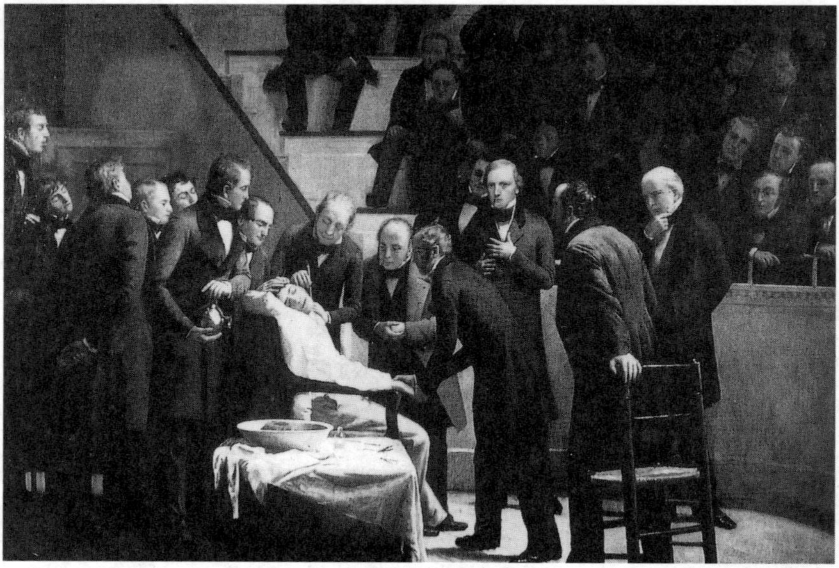

Fig. 1. Demonstration of the first ether narcosis by Morton and Warren, Massachusetts General Hospital, Boston, 16 October 1846

which came some 15 years later. Unfortunately, Semmelweis was obviously often discredited, mainly because of his obsolete scientific approach (Fig. 2) (Thiel 1942). In Vienna, in 1847, shortly after the first narcosis demonstration, he observed the importance of contact infections. As his findings had not been acknowledged in Vienna, he moved to Budapest where he continued his research into fighting contact infection, i.e., puerperal fever, and found full acceptance. Although he was one of the first to discover the secret of sepsis and asepsis – the foundation of modern surgery – he died from sepsis himself on August 1, 1865, mentally affected by progressive paralysis caused by petechial damage to his finger which he incurred while conducting a necropsy. Almost simultaneously, in 1865/66, Joseph Lister published some of the first hints about the importance of antisepsis, preventing wound infection by local chemotherapy (Drees 1989). His practical observations were supported theoretically by Louis Pasteur's description of bacteria in 1863. Schönlein had already created the foundations of bacteriology. Robert Koch took the subject further by cultivating splenitis bacilli in 1877 and detecting the tubercle bacillus in 1882 (Bochalli 1954).

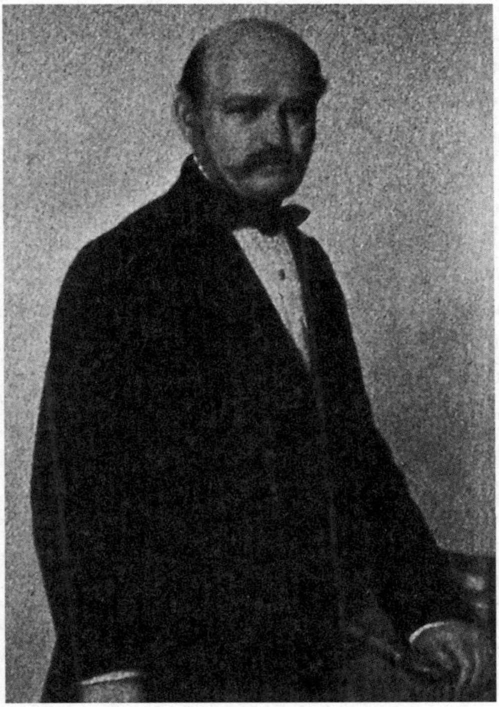

Fig. 2. Ignaz Philipp Semmelweis (1818–1865). Observations on contact infection in Vienna 1847 showed the relationship between sepsis and narcosis

These were the prerequisites and pillars for the development of modern surgery since 1846. However, was there an abrupt change from medieval to modern surgery, or a more gradual development? Have there been any indications of such a change? We cannot answer these questions without analyzing the preceding centuries, in particular 1750–1850, from several points of view, i.e., the medical, social, theological, and political, or even from the viewpoints of the military and of university politics.

Roots of Modern Surgery in Antiquity and the Middle Ages

By the end of the ancient European empires, knowledge about ancient medicine and the art of surgery had been almost lost during the impetuous migration of nations. Western and Middle Europe lapsed into chaos; in Italy several Teutonic tribes engaged in fierce battles. The medical knowledge of those people was a primitive mixture of experience and superstition. Near the turn of the millennium, the Arabs expanded their empire along Southern Europe and North Africa toward the Atlantic. Once they had consolidated their power, the Arabs turned out to be remarkably tolerant toward strangers and people of different faiths. Trade and crafts boomed and delivered an economic basis for art and science, which flourished under Arabic influence. Knowledge of ancient medicine was imparted in Southern Italy at that time by means of Arabic translations and Islam's bridging function between antiquity and the Middle Ages. It was the period of Rhazes, the Persian Galen (850–923), and Avicenna (980–1037), the physician, philosopher and politician who was absorbed in the theories of Aristotle and, from a medical point of view, Hippocrates and Galen; Avicenna's *Canon medicinae* has been the standard medical textbook in Europe for centuries. This made Avicenna Europe's mentor for the medical arts and the successor of the great ancient masters. Abulkasim mainly introduced Alexandrian surgery (Lyons and Petrocelli 1980). All three of these men were strongly influenced by Hippocrates and Galen, on whose work they based their ideas and then imparted that knowledge to others. At that time, by the turn of the millennium, surgery was a part of medicine.

The origins of medieval surgery can be summarized as follows:

- End of ancient European kingdoms: loss of knowledge about ancient medicine during the impetuous migration of nations.
- Islam bridging between antiquity and Middle Ages in Europe.
  a) Rhazes (approx. 850/865–923/925)
  b) Avicenna (980–1037) "Canon Medicinae"
  c) Abulkasim (approx. 912/936/939–1013)
- The origins of European medicine appear to be connected with the Church; the Church represents ancient tradition and preserves civilization.
  a) Surgery as a fringe area of medicine
  b) Just a few non-ecclesiastic, but brilliant exceptions: Salerno, Bologna, Florence, Montpellier

European medicine developed under the influence of the church "representing ancient tradition and preserving civilization" at that time. The church offered safety and continuity for further development. Monks were dedicated to studying ancient sciences such as medicine and rudimentary surgery. The Benedictines promoted medical development. Monte Cassino, their home, was the center that influenced other monasteries such as St. Gallen, St Rupert at Salzburg, Fulda, Tours, the Lake Constance island of Reichenau and finally even St. Kilian in Würzburg. Monastic medicine was promoted by monasteries and cathedral chapter schools with the support of the church in Italy, France and Southern Germany. The church monopolized scientific education, including medicine. Due to the dominance of the Benedictines in every field of science, medicine was strongly influenced by the clergy. There were no major surgical activities without clerical control.

One exception should be mentioned, however: in Salerno, close to Naples, only 150 km away from Monte Cassino, a guild of physicians called "civitas hippocratica" conserved the ancient tradition. Salerno's open-minded and tolerant attitude attracted many from various faiths who were interested in medical science. Confronted with that prototype of a university, a great surgical personality, Roger Frugardi, appeared during the twelfth century (Keil 1995; Gurlt 1898). He was a Lombard who created a medical-surgical school which spread across Europe. He mastered, taught and demonstrated several surgical procedures, such as trepanation, intestinal anastomoses, stabilization of bone fractures and wound dressing, to name a few. Roger Frugardi, a surgeon 800 years ago, contributed new findings and imparted much ancient surgical knowledge. With his mixture of existing and new experience, he brought surgery at that time to a peak. The systematic work attributed to him deeply influenced surgery in Europe. Wherever surgeons worked, from Flanders and Paris to Sicily, they followed their master, Roger of Salerno. This was even true in the universities of Bologna, Parma, and Montpellier.

Separation of Surgery from Medical Science in the Middle Ages

Until the Middle Ages, the authorities had not clearly separated surgery from scientific medicine. Surgery had been, however, a special branch in their characteristic disagreement with theoretic medical sciences: the surgeon believed in and acted according to what he saw. The physician, however, believed in and acted according to medical and mostly theoretical principles. Since the twelfth century, the clergy and, thus, most medical practitioners, were forbidden to deal with surgical activities, especially since the edict of Tours. The church abhorred blood and, consequently, surgery. Surgical education was banished from medical schools and surgical literature at medical faculties was reduced. This was due not only to clerical influence but also to the "Zeitgeist", the particular medieval mentality also called scholasticism. This trend prevailed at the early universities established for the instruction of the clergy. Under the influence of the church, universities developed, aiming toward the stabilization and incontestability of ecclesiastic dogmas using the traditional knowledge of great ancient thinkers, such as Hippocrates (460–377 b.c.) or Galen (129–198/201 a.d.). This scholastic method aspired to bring religious dogma into line with ancient science. This mentality was also a consequence of the balance of clerical and secular power, which did not always favor the church. Scholastic science was merely theoretical. There was a constant quarrel with ecclesiastical institutions. The principle of authority and assimilation was observed and taught no more than reading, translation and dialectic critical interpretation of ancient and Arabic authors (with Galen's theory on the humors of the body prevailing). Scholasticism considered practical activities, such as surgery, as of inferior value and degrading for university men. The ban on surgical activity was accepted, with regional variations: Teoderico di Borgognoni was among the best surgeons during the 1250s and was a Dominican friar and officiating bishop of Cervia; Guy de Chauliac, the best surgeon of the 1350s, belonged to the cathedral chapter and was a private chaplain of the Pope; in the diocese of Würzburg, however, members of the clergy were periodically excluded as spectators from surgical operations.

The separation of surgery from medical science can thus be summarized as follows:

- 1163 Council of Tours: clerics are no longer allowed to engage in surgical matters.
- As a consequence of that Council:
  a) Surgical instruction is banished from medical schools.
  b) Surgical literature disappears from university faculties.
- Scholasticism intensifies this influence:
  a) Dogmatism, credulity in authorities.
  b) Scholastic science restricted to theory.

With this drastic division, surgery was separated from medicine or, as described more vividly by Detlev Rüster (1986), "not between medicine and surgery, but neatly across surgery itself – its theory and practice" (Rüster 1993). Surgery was still taught by universities but practical reference and application were lacking.

This cleared the field for non-academic practitioners, the workman-like healers who had existed earlier and who continued their activity unrivaled by academics. In addition to ideological and theological reasons, practical medical education appeared much too expensive and was neither demanded nor promoted by the authorities.

Protagonists of Medieval and Early Modern Surgery

Nevertheless, we know of several outstanding personalities of various origins who were well reputed surgeons (Table 1). Roger of Parma, in the twelfth century, has been mentioned already. Influenced by the school of Salerno and by his own experience, he stated that suppuration does not favor wound healing at all, but should be prevented. Influenced by the school of Bologna and Parma in Lombardy, several other important surgeons were being formed by a full scientific university education, in which surgery and medicine were still considered together.

Ugo of Lucca (1155–1200) was against the general opinion that suppuration would favor wound healing. His method of avoiding suppuration and accelerating wound healing consisted of keeping the physician and patient, the tools and dressing mate-

TABLE 1. Personages in medieval surgery

Personage	Period	School	Status	Place of activity
From Italy				
Rogerio filius Frugardi	1140–1195	University	Barber-surgeon	Parma
Ugo da Lucca	1155–1200	University	Barber-surgeon	Southern Italy
Guglielmo da Saliceto	1201–1277	University	Barber-surgeon	Bologna
Lanfranchi of Milan	1245–1306	University	Barber-surgeon	Milan Paris
From France				
Henri de Mondeville	1260–1325	University	Surgeon in ordinary	Paris
Guy de Chauliac	1300–1368	University	Physician Surgeon Surgeon	Lyon Avignon Paris
Ambroise Paré	1510–1590	Handicraft	Surgeon, military physician in ordinary	Paris
Jacques Beaulieu	1651–1719	Handicraft	Cutter of calculus	Paris, Europe
Jean Dominique Larrey	1766–1842	Handicraft	Military physician in ordinary	Paris
From Flanders				
Andreas Vesalius	1514–1564	University	Anatomist, physician, surgeon, royal ordinary	Padua Brussels Madrid
From Germany				
Hanns v. Gersdorff	1455–1529	Handicraft	Barber-surgeon	Strasbourg
Caspar Stromayr	1510–1567	Handicraft	Barber-surgeon	Lindau
Georg Bartisch	1535–1607	Handicraft	Surgeon in ordinary	Dresden
Wilhelm Fabry of Hilden	1560–1634	Handicraft	Barber-surgeon	Southern Germany
Lorenz Heister	1683–1758	University	Physician	Altdorf

rials, and the injuries themselves, meticulously clean with alcohol dressings. Nowadays this observation has become an accepted matter of fact but at that time only his disciples Bruno of Longoburgo and Teoderico of Cervia accepted it as a doctrine.

Guglielmo di Saliceto (1210–1275), also at Bologna, is one of the Lombard surgeons who rediscovered an interest in human anatomy as a prerequisite for successful surgery.

The last great surgeon of Lombard provenance was Lanfranchi of Milan (1245–1306), Guglielmo di Saliceto's disciple at Bologna, who pushed medieval Italian surgery to its highest peak. As a follower of the Emperor, he was deported from Milan in 1295 and moved to Lyon, later to Paris. There, in the new stronghold of surgery, he found excellent conditions and royal support for completing his great manual of surgery.

Provençal physicians and Flemish surgeons became the new leaders of surgery, in particular Henri de Mondeville (1250/1260–1320/1325) of Hermundsweil in Normandy (lecturing at Kosmas college in Paris, a surgical, university-like medical school) and, later, Guy de Chauliac (1300–1368), personal surgeon to three popes at Avignon. Chauliac's manual *Chirurgia magna* (1363) was the standard for surgical education and practice until early modern times, rivaled only by the great Flemish surgeon Yperman and by Schelling during the fourteenth century.

Despite these men, surgical practice was pushed out of universities and practicing surgeons were mostly recruited from craftsmen. In Paris in 1295 the medical faculty of the Sorbonne, with no surgical practice, coexisted with an academic college for surgeons. Lanfranchi had connections there. Yperman, Schelling and Mondeville frequented it for surgical training. Lanfranchi presented the abundance of scientific surgery to the surgeons of Paris, thus shifting the leadership in surgery from Italy to France between the years 1295 and 1300. At that time, practical surgery split off from scientific medicine, shaking off its scholastic chains. The surgical college of Kosmas, structured scholastically by Mondeville, where lectures were given in Latin, was confirmed by the king and considered almost equal in rank with the university, against the strong opposition of the Sorbonne.

Ambroise Paré (1510–1590) had not studied at the Collège de St Côme, but he should be considered one of the great surgeons of France (Fig. 3). He began as a barber's apprentice and continued his education with the wound dressers of the Paris hos-

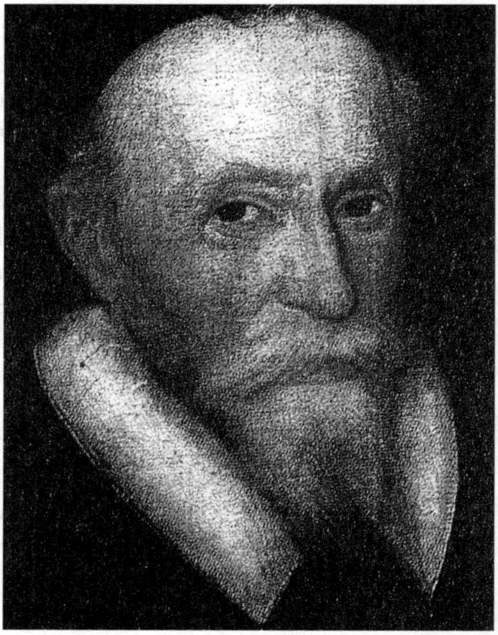

Fig. 3. Ambroise Paré (1510–1590), "the surgeon of France", physician in ordinary to the king

pital, Hôtel-Dieu. He joined the French army in 1536 and became famous for his method of almost painless wound treatment: instead of boiling oil he applied a special pain-alleviating tincture. He published this procedure in his manual *The Treatment of Bullet Wounds* in 1545, and the army showered him with glory. The following anecdote will help us to understand. During the siege of Metz, Paré sneaked through the enemy lines by order of the king. When he arrived in town, the soldiers exclaimed "We won't die, even when wounded. Paré is in our midst!"

Military surgeons of the powerful French kings had a good reputation. Paré became personal physician to the king and, as a distinguished master surgeon, was admitted to the venerable Collège de St Côme. He never forgot to remain modest, however, as this statement shows: "I dressed his wound, God healed him."

By the end of the Middle Ages, some German surgeons also rose from among the military surgeons. Yperman and Schelling, from the fourteenth century, have been mentioned already. Hanns von Gersdorff (1455–1529) originated from Alsace. He had a solid surgical craftsman's education and gathered experience during his travels. Then, qualified as a military surgeon during

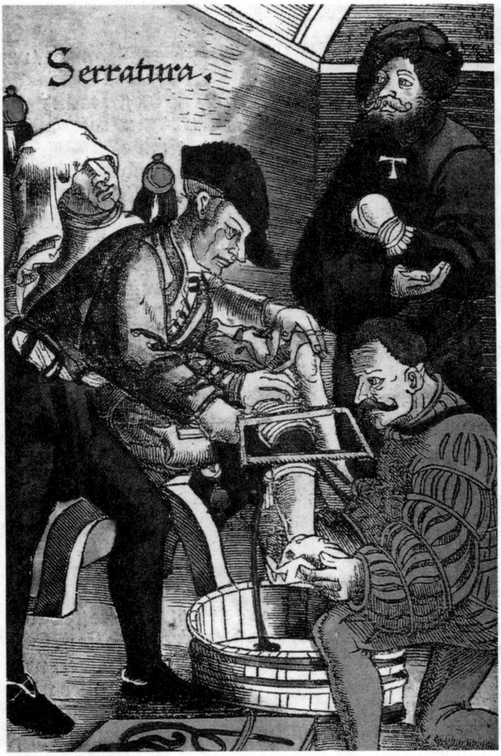

Fig. 4. Illustration of an amputation in the *Feldtbuch der Wundartzney 1540* by Hanns von Gersdorff (1455–1529)

the wars against Charles the Bold of Burgundy (1476/77), he finally became surgeon at Strasbourg, where he wrote his book on military surgery entitled *Feldtbuch der Wundtartzney* (1517). Luckily, Johannes von Gutenberg's movable type already existed for its dissemination. The craftsman-surgeon had chosen the best medium to impart his knowledge and experience to younger colleagues (Fig. 4). His craftsmanship did not prevent Hanns von Gersdorff from constantly mentioning the influences which had produced his ideas and activities. So he lauded the shining example of Guy de Chauliac and was interested in the "sleeping sponge" Chauliac had developed – a debated method of narcotizing patients and easing pain. Certainly this was an early step toward later narcosis. Gersdorff also mentioned Avicenna, Abulkasim, Roger Frugardi and others who had influenced medieval surgery.

Caspar Stromayr (about 1510–1567) also figures among craftsmen-surgeons. He became known through a richly illus-

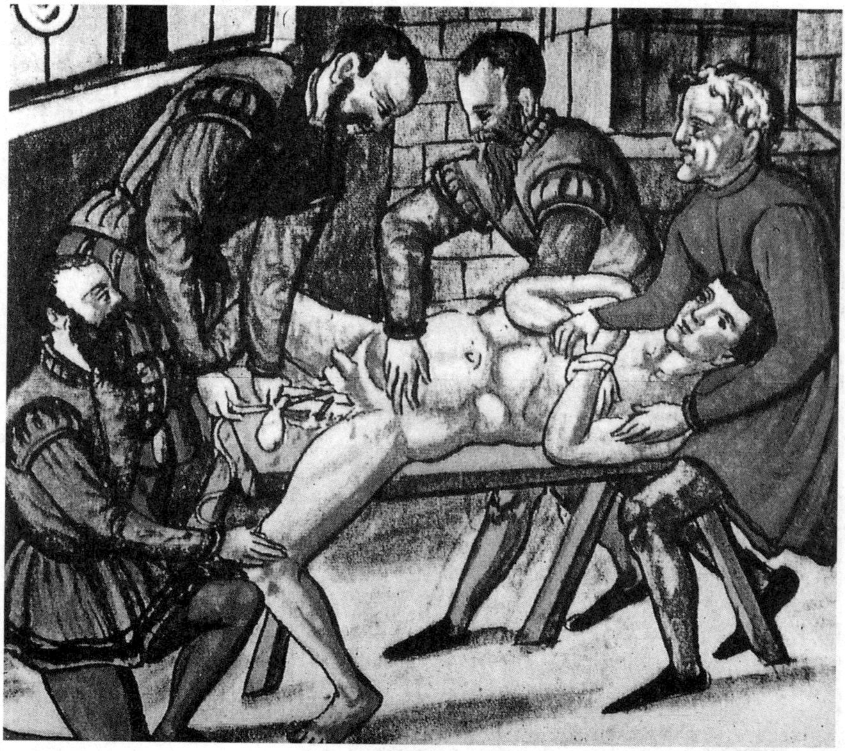

Fig. 5. Caspar Strohmayr (1510–1567). Operating manual with colored illustrations, 1559. Inguinal hernia surgery

trated surgical text book compiled in 1559, in which he brilliantly described every possible surgical technique in a series of figures (Fig. 5). He was the first to differentiate between the direct and indirect inguinal hernia and, even before Bassini's radical technique, to surgically repair testicular hernia, saving the testes. This book is regarded as an occult work, similar to that by Heinrich von Pfolspeundt entitled *Bündth-Ertzney* (medication of wounds) compiled around 1460, in which he was the first to describe the tube pedicle method for skin transplantation as well as his experience during the battle against the Polish army.

Paracelsus (1494–1541), the famous antimedical and eminent authority of medieval Southern Germany, vehemently criticized the surgical profession. This description characterizes the reputation of many a surgeon at the time: "The surgeon should not be a whoremonger, hangman, apostate or a 'sky pilot'" (Sud-

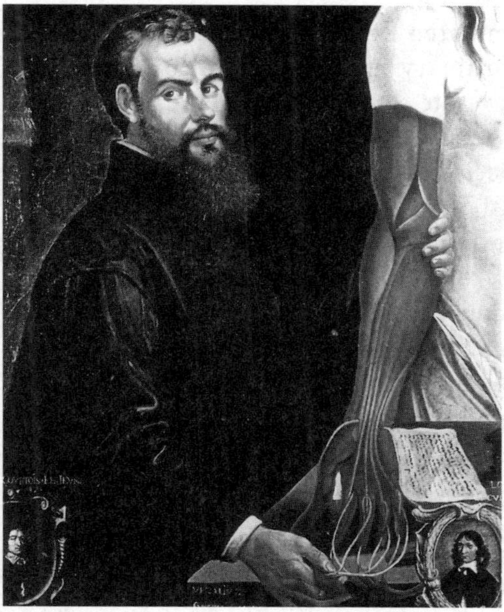

Fig. 6. Andreas Vesal (1514–1564), physician in ordinary to Emperor Charles V

hoff 1936; Pächter 1955). He suggested, however, a course schedule for surgeons consisting of the complete anatomy, pharmacy, operative techniques and methods of wound healing.

During the sixteenth century and as a consequence of the Renaissance mentality with its revival of ancient origins, a new star appeared: Andreas Vesalius (Andries van Wesel, 1514–1564) from Brussels (Schott 1996; Fig. 6), who studied at Leuven, Paris and Padua. He dissected mainly human corpses and thus greatly surpassed Galen's basic anatomic knowledge gained from animal dissections. At the early age of 23 he became professor of anatomy and surgery at Padua University with its proverbial liberty, Libertas Pataviana. The university of Padua had been founded in 1222 by discontented students and professors from Bologna. Vesalius's anatomic medical observations often contrasted with those of Galen, whose medical authority had not been questioned until the beginning of the Renaissance. Due to his fame, Vesalius became personal physician to the emperor Charles V and later followed him to Spain. His life ended for unknown reasons during a journey to Palestine in 1564.

The famous early modern physician Georg Bartisch (1535–1607), born in Dresden as son of a barber, was apprenticed to wound healers and accumulated experience in the treatment of wounds. He was oculist in ordinary to the electoral court and surgeon at Dresden in 1558. He wrote a remarkable manual on surgery; however, it was never published, due to the Elector's lack of interest. Nevertheless, Bartisch personally organized the publication of the first German textbook on ophthalmology.

Another important German surgeon was Wilhelm Fabry von Hilden (1560–1634). After his surgical apprenticeship in Switzerland and Southern Germany he made several important contributions to surgery. Military surgeons relied upon his experience and followed his instructions for their equipment, the so-called "cista militaris". Navy surgeons used to carry with them at least one of his books. His knowledge qualified him as a "German Paré", but the political situation was different. Germany was not a centralized nation but consisted of various territorial governments. Therefore, there were only faint signs of German surgery until the time of Matthäus Gottfried Purmann (1648–1711).

Three Characters Representative of the Turning Point

The following three personalities perhaps symbolize the dazzling variety of surgery at different levels and stages of development:

- The journeyman cutter of calculus, Jacques Beaulieu (1651–1719): from a quack doctor to a studious practitioner
- The military surgeon, Jean Dominique Larrey (1766–1842): the personification of the military surgeon
- The university surgeon, Lorenz Heister (1683–1758): the pioneer of scientific surgery in Germany

Jacques Beaulieu

Jacques Beaulieu (1651–1719) is considered one of the most adventurous and dazzling characters in the history of medicine and represents the typical so-called "surgeon" of his time. He was born in Burgundian Besançon in 1651. He started his career as a private soldier who could not reach officers' rank because of his poor background. Then he assisted an Italian hernia and stone cutter, which was equally important. Consequently, a lot of patients who could not find help from the official physicians (physici, medici) felt convinced by the "master's" impressive leaflets announcing the arrival of the world-famous "hernieur" and "inciseur de la pierre." The "world-famous master" used to perform his surgery, depending on circumstances, either in his own booth or on an inn table, or he simply fastened the patient to a cart in the center of the village, with the most dubious chance of success. At nightfall, the booth was quickly taken apart, leaving the patient to a most uncertain fate. The following story depicts his commercial skill. Being a simple country lad without any recognized education, he was not lacking in ambition and self-confidence, qualities that are necessary for puffing. He risked all and appeared in a monk's habit in Paris in 1697, beginning to play his successful role as "Frère Jacques". This was to suggest to people his high vocation, divine blessing and knowledge of the good old monastic medicine. He was able to evoke the interest of a prince's personal physician and was allowed to perform a successful stone-cutting in public under the control of physicians. This was his breakthrough and he was admitted to operate at the Hôtel-Dieu and the Charité in Paris, where the physicians did not like the idea at all. However, his successes did not continue and one night he had to leave Paris clandestinely, but as a rich man. "Friar Jacob" was able to learn from his own mistakes. He detected the disadvantages of his method and improved it, possibly influenced by his contact with the famous medical school of Leiden. He no longer placed his knife perineally at random but laterally, thus avoiding damage to the urethra and sphincter. That "sectio lateralis" encouraged Gerhard van Swieten, the famous physician in Vienna and disciple of Boerhaeve, who was the "pope" of medicine at Leiden, to state that Friar Jacob had learnt from his mistakes and that, later in France, he had been much more successful with lateral herniotomy.

The career of Jacques Beaulieu, "Friar Jacob", symbolizes the development of fifteenth and sixteenth century surgery, "from the abysses of ignorance and adventure to an honest job".

Jean Dominique Larrey (1766–1842)

"Eyes like a hawk, hands like a virgin with a lion-hearted courage": so Detlef Rüster (1986) described military surgeons like the exemplary Jean Dominique Larrey. Larrey's surgical and military career was linked with the French revolution and Napoleon. Later, Larrey would become Napoleon's personal physician and a senior military surgeon. Napoleon called him "the boldest man I ever got to know". Thus, during the Battle of Borodino, where there were many losses, he performed more than 200 amputations overnight. Larrey was the most prominent military surgeon of his time. He was convinced of the American concept of early amputation to prevent infection. Following the example of German *Landsknecht-Truppen* (paid soldiers), he also introduced "ambulances volantes", quickly maneuverable ambulance units which searched for injured soldiers at the very front line to give them first aid. He was the surgeon-in-chief of those "flying ambulances" (Fig. 7). This concept of flying ambulances is admirable for two reasons: (1) quick surgical treatment of injuries was achieved, before infection threatened survival; and (2) the injured were prevented from being taken prisoner or given the coup de grâce by the enemy.

Larrey himself wrote: "The mere sight of flying ambulances following the avant-garde increased the army's confidence and courage in fight."

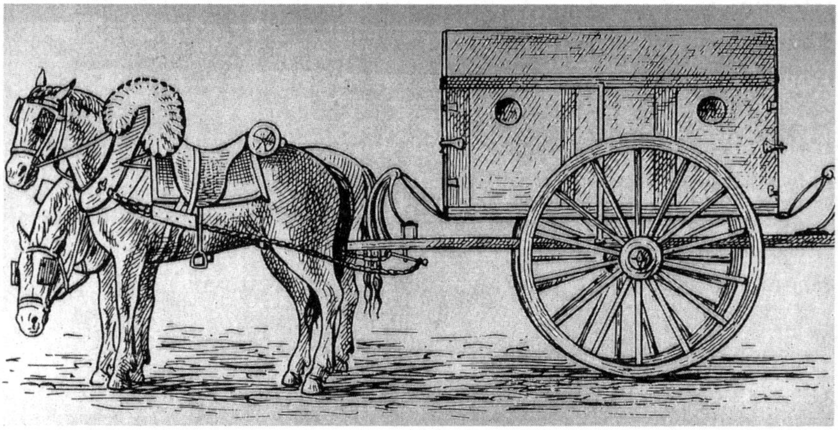

Fig. 7. Larrey's flying ambulances

Additionally, he organized a special unit to transport the injured further back in their own lines, to military hospitals, thus enormously increasing their chance of survival. Let us consider some numbers. The Napoleonic wars called for a new size of army: 94,000 soldiers followed Napoleon to the battle near Austerlitz where he lost 12,000. Near Smolensk, 20,000 out of 180,000 died. Not even half of 600,000 soldiers returned from the campaign in Russia. More than 30,000 of 72,000 men died near Waterloo. From 1792 to 1815, the French army numbered 4.5 million soldiers, 2.5 million of whom were killed, but only 150,000 directly on the battle field. Most men died before or after the fighting, during long marches with insufficient equipment and in a state of physical exhaustion. Among those huge armies, epidemics such as dysentery, marsh fever, typhus and skin diseases raged horribly and terrible wound infection was described in various reports. Larrey's reputation among the soldiers is illustrated by the following story. During the Beresina retreat, Larrey continued rushing over the bridge to help the injured until he himself fainted with exhaustion. Passing soldiers recognized him and carried him to the bridge. Whenever they could not go on, they handed him to the men in front and shouted, "This is Larrey". Notwithstanding their fear of death, Larrey was passed from hand to hand over the bridge to the other bank, always accompanied by the call, "This is Larrey!". Napoleon himself, however, had to free his way with guns.

Lorenz Heister
(1683–1758, Fig. 8)

At Leiden, Jacques Beaulieu met the later star of German surgery, Lorenz Heister, who was born in Frankfurt and died in Helmstedt (Geiger 1983; Korff 1975). Heister was as young as 14 when Frère Jacques started his Paris adventure. Heister's own education was completely different. He began to study medicine in 1702 at Giessen, Amsterdam and Leiden, where, as a disciple of the master surgeon Jan Jacob Rau, he probably met Jacques Beaulieu, Frère Jacques, whom he regarded rather critically at that time.

Rau's surgical and anatomical school was not confined to theory, but he also taught practical surgery to Lorenz Heister, who was deeply impressed by his professor. During the summer

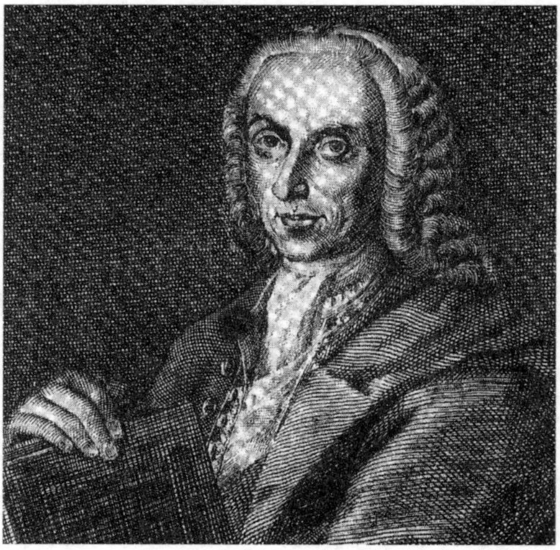

Fig. 8. Lorenz Heister (1683–1758), "the university surgeon"

campaigns between 1707 and 1710, Heister periodically interrupted his studies to gain practical experience as a military surgeon. He received his medical doctor's degree in 1708 and from 1709 he lectured in anatomy and surgery at Dutch universities. At the age of 27 he was offered a chair of anatomy, surgery and botany at the University of Altdorf, near Nuremberg, and gave his inaugural lecture in 1710. Heister was a surgeon, not the usual craftsman, but with an academic background in theory and practice. He represented much of what we regard as the modern surgeon. His colleagues mostly gave theoretical lectures but scorned practical application, which was considered the task of craftsmen-surgeons. This was not so for Lorenz Heister. He was in fact the first German university surgeon. He initiated the turning point at which surgery gradually became incorporated into scientific university medicine. It was quite a novel type of procedure to offer him a German university chair, a rarity in Europe. He was the first high-ranking academic surgeon. At Altdorf, he became a distinguished scientist who promoted practical work. His manual on surgery, *Chirurgie*, was published in Nuremberg in 1719 and represents the knowledge taught at that time. His unique achievement was the rehabilitation of surgery as a science, setting standards for surgeons all over Europe. The University of Helmstedt offered him a chair exclusively for surgery. Due to his knowledge of anatomy, he was able to perform suprapubic cystotomy, "sectio alta", a standard surgical procedure which is still practiced nowadays. His career was at the peak; he was a successful physician and surgeon, an acknowledged scientist full of merit. When Heister died in 1758 he had led surgery out of the Dark Ages toward the "century of surgeons" which started in 1850 (Thorwald 1972). Heister had reached his goal in life: to combine practical surgery with university medicine and science. More major efforts than one person's glory, however, were needed to raise the reputation of surgery as a whole.

Importance of Non-academic Surgery Before 1850

Until the beginning of the nineteenth century, there were on the one hand academic physicians consulted by the aristocracy, royal households, higher-ranking clergy, and wealthy town citizens (about 10% of the population), with, on the other, a non-uniform group of craftsmen healers. The latter included resident corporate barber-surgeons, traveling experts in surgery (lithotomists, herniotomists, cataract needlers, dentists), and army surgeons, but there were also quacks and fraudsters. The craftsmen healers were competent enough to treat middle-class citizens, craftsmen, large farmers and the lower-ranking clergy (about 25% of the population). The lower classes (65% of the population) used to consult lay healers who asked for little or no money (Probst 1992). Only those patients who could afford the high fees used to consult "real" physicians for internal and quite exclusively conservative medicine. The physicians ranked first in the health hierarchy and were largely autonomous. Their reputation was not based, however, on successful treatment, but more on their academic education and their resulting social position. In addition, the number of physicians did not meet the demand, especially in the countryside. The enormous gaps in medical care were left for non-academic healers in surgery and obstetrics to fill. The group of non-academic healers was inhomogeneous, consisting of professionals and laymen. The particular impact of non-academic healers was due to their social proximityto a major part of the population and the much lower fees they asked.

Everyday life for surgeons before the nineteenth century can thus be summarized as follows:

1. Medical supply and demand by groups:
   - Physicians: aristocracy, royal households, higher ranking clergy, town citizens (10%)
   - Barber-surgeons: middle class (craftsmen) citizens, major farmers, lower ranking clergy (25%)
   - Lay healers: lower classes (65%)
2. Non-uniform class of surgeons:
   - Resident, corporate barber-surgeons
   - Traveling experts in surgery
   - Army surgeons
   - Quacks and defrauders

What were the prerequisites for surgery to be reintegrated into academic and scientific medicine, an inevitable condition for the new era of surgery since 1850?

The existence of several extraordinary surgical pioneers such as Lorenz Heister should not obscure the state of surgery during the eighteenth century. The education and activity of those personalities had been totally dissimilar and their reputation was low, with some few exceptions (Drees 1989). This was noticed by the authorities and, under the influence of physicians and personal surgeons (even according to the requirements of military health), they planned to change the situation. While in France surgical schools existed much earlier (such as the Collège de St. Côme, which had the same status as the university from 1743), in Germany this development started reluctantly and much later, as can be seen by the examples of Berlin in Prussia and Vienna in Austria (Table 2).

Gentle Approach Due to Military Obligations

When we consider what influenced the development of surgery during the seventeenth and eighteenth century, a lack of surgical care in military health is apparent. The losses due to bad health before battles appeared much higher than those suffered during battle. The death rate caused by poor surgical care of injuries exceeds, by far, the direct victims. The small number, bad training and insufficient equipment of military barber-sur-

TABLE 2. Better education by specialized surgical schools

France	Pioneering: Collège de St. Côme
Berlin	Foundation of the *Theatrum anatomicum* by Holtzendorff in 1713, enlarged in 1723 to form the *Collegium medico-chirurgicum* offering extensive training The Charité Hospital set up in 1727 as a practical training center
Vienna	Medical surgical school in 1781, Josephs-Akademie in 1785
Prussia etc.	Progressive legislation regulating training and position of physicians during the eighteenth and nineteenth century, top-ranking in Prussia

geons, as well as inadequate transport of the injured, was recognized by two Prussian senior military surgeons, Gehema and Purmann, who explained it to their sovereign. Military surgeons and sovereigns agreed about the deplorable state of affairs, claiming to improve them mainly by an academic education for surgeons, but for different motives: the sovereign wished to increase his army's fighting strength; the surgeons – we think so, at least – intended to take care of the individual patient, the fellow-Christian. The growing armies required quick decisions. Around 1630, the Prussian army had 11,000 soldiers, during wartime 38 500. The "soldier king", Frederick William I, handed on to his son, Frederick the Great (reign 1740–1786), more than 80,000 men under arms; during war time, however, he mobilized up to 218,000. This rearmament required more surgeons and more education for them.

Ernst Conrad von Holtzendorff (1688–1751), Frederick William's senior military physician, succeeded in proposing to the king's "tobacco assembly" the foundation of a "theatrum anatomicum" and a chair of military surgery in Berlin in 1713. Under his influence, this became a "collegium medico-chirurgicum" (Havig 1990), thus laying the foundations of a scientific-theoretical school of surgeons, especially military surgeons. The training program consisted of anatomy, Latin, internal medicine and natural scientific disciplines such as botany. An examination concluded this education. Scientific education at the collegium medico-chirurgicum represented an essential requirement for the fur-

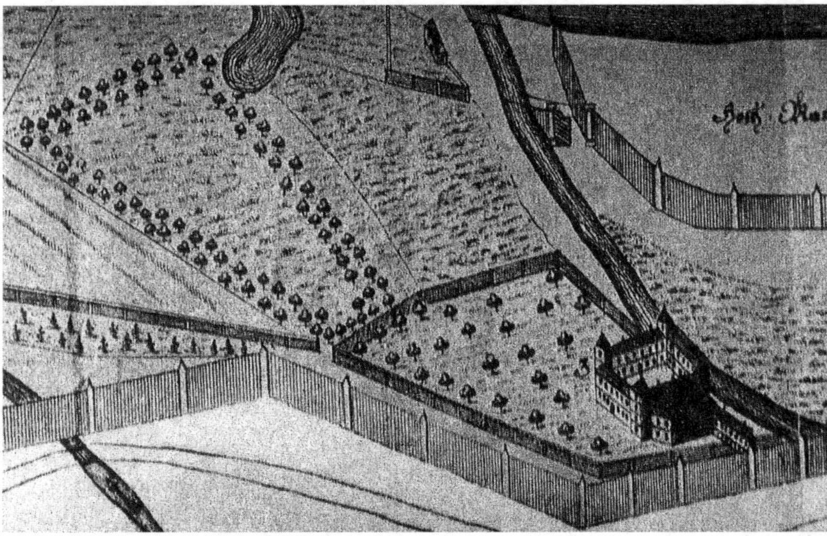

Fig. 9. The plague hospital in Berlin in 1727, the future Charité

ther development of surgery and its reintegration into academic medicine. For practical training, the king chose a former plague hospital, later called the Charité (Fig. 9). In this way, Holtzendorff's idea of unifying surgery and internal medicine in a common practical training center was realized. The hospital was opened on January 1, 1727. Later it would become the most prominent center for German medicine and surgery.

Many a famous surgeon and military surgeon lectured or studied at the Charité. Johann Anton Christian Theden (1714–1797), in particular, pursued the path laid down by Holtzendorff. He became the first brigadier-general of the surgical corps in 1786. He even succeeded in separating surgeons from barbers, thus discharging surgeons from the task of shaving all staff members once a week. He also abolished the term "Feldscher", which meant "army-surgeon". Similar trends can be observed in France with the foundation of the Academie de Chirurgie in 1731, which finally gained university rank in 1794. In Vienna, at the time of Emperor Joseph II, a medical-surgical school was founded in 1781 that generated the Josephs-Akademie in 1785 (Skopec 1990). The latter, also called Josephinum, was entitled to confer doctors' and masters' degrees at the university level and its graduates alone were allowed to be military surgeons.

Legal Steps to Regulate Public Health

Parallel to this development the sovereigns regulated public health by territorial law. In Brandenburg-Prussia, public health gained new importance through the Great Elector's Medizinaledikt (edict of health) in 1685 (Fischer 1965). That edict and its later supplements (the first in 1693) contained instructions for physicians, pharmacists, barbers and midwives. A list of fees was established and professional duties were prescribed. A substantially enlarged edition was published in 1725. This was the first subdivision of the medical profession according to different qualifications: three ranks of academic physicians, two ranks of *Wundärzte* (an obsolete term for surgeons: wound doctors) or town and country surgeons. Drastic modifications were added in 1811 and 1825. Surgeons were distinguished from barbers. The system of town and country surgeons was replaced by first- and second-rank surgeons. First-rank surgeons had to graduate at a partly academic surgical school. Second-rank surgeons had their craftsman instruction as before. This legislation for the medical profession was adopted by many smaller German territories. In the civil and military field, one could observe that surgeons were better qualified due to a better academic education and specialization in their surgical activity and to their freedom from other service duties. This was the way for surgeons to go to be reintegrated into scientific medicine. This development was in fact achieved in Prussia in 1852, when legislation required physicians of every discipline (including surgeons), to graduate at a medical school before they were entitled to exercise their profession. The former mere surgical schools gradually disappeared, being incorporated into universities. The reintegration of surgery into academic medicine between 1750 and 1850 was decisive in preparing the way for modern surgery.

Reintegration of Surgery: A Political and Social Problem

In Germany Lorenz Heister paved the way for surgery as a university discipline, becoming its first full university professor. His studies and contributions to coordinating medicine and surgery were still well regarded during the eighteenth century. But

Table 3. University surgery

Lorenz Heister paved the way for university surgery	Discussions in every field of academic life
Final union, but still problematic politically and socially	Inaugural address of Matthäus von Mederer und Wuthwehr (surgeon at Freiburg 1773–1796)
Practical surgery integrated in universities	"Surgeon of the North": August Gottlieb Richter at Göttingen (1766–1803)
	"Surgeon of the South": Carl Caspar von Siebold at Würzburg (1769–1807)

the discussion intensified; by the end of the eighteenth century the chair of surgery, anatomy and obstetrics came into existence, with practical applications (Kilian 1980). Year by year, more students received clinical instruction in surgery. There was no more separation between the two branches. University departments for internal medicine and surgery developed. The increase in scientific surgical research was manifested by the foundation of numerous periodicals: surgery had gained ground at universities (Table 3).

In contrast to those highly educated university surgeons, however, there were hosts of quack doctors. Various medical regulations on education, examinations and descriptions of titles did not improve the general confusion. The universities produced fewer skilled surgeons than were needed and had to compete with military surgical academies on the French model, a most unpleasant feature which made the traditional separation seem more acceptable.

This background explains why coordinating internal medicine and surgery within the common profession of physician was mainly a social and political problem. Organizational problems aggravated the situation.

A consequent coordination of both professions finally seemed to mean that , on the one hand, graduate physicians had to do much of the former surgeon's job and, on the other hand, many an untrained surgeon would profit from the privileges of a physician.

The discussion penetrated academic life, papers in journals, doctoral theses, and encyclopedias. Encyclopedias enjoyed great popularity during the eighteenth century and in their collection of medical science the head word "surgery" covered several columns about the separation of surgery from academic internal medicine and the extent of its re-coordination. Inaugural lectures often seemed political issues. One of them, and its concomitant scandal, even became medical history (Rüster 1993). The 34-year-old professor of surgery, Matthäus Mederer von Mederer und Wuthwehr, received a call to Freiburg/Breisgau in 1773. After his normal apprenticeship, Mederer had become a fully trained and successful army surgeon and was appointed professor by Empress Maria Theresia. His inaugural lecture "About the necessity of re-coordinating both branches, surgery and internal medicine" was heavily contested by students and professors who shouted him down. They felt insulted by his statement that both branches were equivalent. However, in his initial address to the audience, he had emphasized that no diplomatic compliments should be expected, as he had been "brought up to the sound of weapons." This introduction was followed by his vehement criticism of the church for being responsible for the split during the thirteenth century; a really bold statement in the conservative Austrian town of Freiburg.

The audience was boiling with rage when Mederer pointed out once again "that the theory of medicine and surgery was just the same and, therefore, the common base of medical art. Surgery required even more than theoretic knowledge, that is manual skill." Accordingly, Mederer proposed "that every physician should have been a surgeon before being admitted to clinical practice. A physician might stay with clinical practice until his sharp eye and his steady hand will decrease with growing age." He concluded that both university disciplines could peacefully coexist that way: "However certain snakes, the scum of arrogance, continue to prevent the access to higher perfection of sciences. May that vermin let surgery unmolested!" Whoever was opposed to an equal status for surgery felt directly insulted, of course.

With this inaugural lecture Mederer demonstrated the tough conflict but also the fast and irresistible progress of surgeons. When he left Freiburg in 1796, his students honored him with a serenade and the faculty conferred on him the title of "diplomatic doctor of medicine". He was ennobled like other academic surgeons and died as a most respectable man in Vienna in 1805.

PRACTICAL SURGERY REACHES GERMAN UNIVERSITIES

As mentioned before, tempers ran high over the question of coordinating surgery with internal medicine. This did not change until the 1850s. The subject of discussion, however, was the status of less-trained surgeons not that of well-established prominent scientific surgeons.

Two surgical personalities appeared on the university scene near the end of the eighteenth century, Carl Caspar von Siebold at Würzburg and August Gottlieb Richter at Göttingen, who established important schools (Fig. 10). In analogy to Carl Caspar von Siebold, the "surgeon of the south", August Gottlieb Richter was the "surgeon of the north". He succeeded the excellent surgeon Albrecht von Haller in the chair of surgery. Remarkably, Albrecht von Haller, who was the author of several famous surgical textbooks and encyclopedias (most importantly *Bibliotheca botanica, chirurgica anatomica* and *Medicinae practicae*) never personally performed surgery on a living patient. While he was professor of surgery from 1736 until 1753 at Göttingen he still followed the old tradition, giving his instructions for operations to one of his assistant surgical directors during the training of students.

When August Gottlieb Richter accepted this famous chair in 1766, the effect was similar to that of Carl Caspar von Siebold in Würzburg. He gave many most interesting lectures on surgery, ophthalmology and special therapy as well as providing clinical training in the hospital. His major objective was for surgery and internal medicine to coexist as equals. He succeeded in founding a surgical department at Göttingen in 1781. He was the enthusiastic author of 15 surgical volumes; his two volumes on hernias are famous and fundamental. When he died on 23 July 1812, he left many disciples, one of whom was C. J. M. von Langenbeck, uncle of Bernhard von Langenbeck, whose school generated many surgeons.

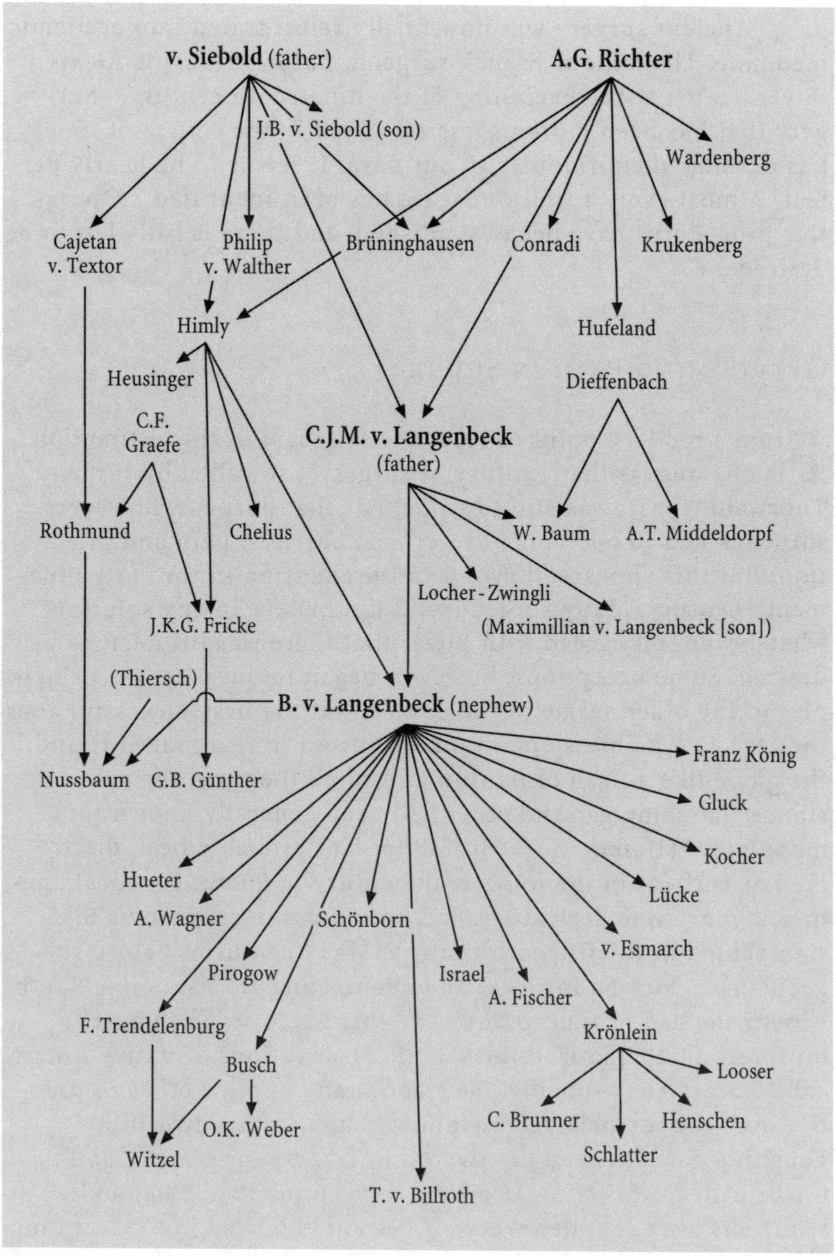

Fig. 10. Family trees of S. Richter (Göttingen) and C.C. v. Siebold (Würzburg)

Ancient surgery was now finally reintegrated into academic medicine. The famous French surgeon, Baron Professor Alexis Boyer, stated at the beginning of the nineteenth century, "Surgery that has been more or less exercised in the course of times has developed enormously in our days. It seems to be nearly perfect. Almost every surgical disease has been identified... Operative procedures have been established, and there is little left to be desired... ."

32 Overcoming Pain in Surgery

From a modern point of view, the falseness of this estimation is obvious, as the "century of surgery", so called by Jürgen Thorwald (1972), was still to come. For that purpose, however, surgeons had to overcome two crucial barriers: pain and infection. But this appeared beyond comprehension in the early nineteenth century. Many surgeons did not believe in any solution whatsoever and agreed with Boyer that there was little left to be desired. Some exceptions, however, began to question the principles of the older surgery. The news about the first successful anesthesia, i.e., a painless operation, in Boston in 1846, raced round the globe like a flash of lightning. And all the time, the substances laughing gas and ether had been generally known for many years (Haferkamp 1989). Ether had probably been discovered as early as in the fourteenth century in Spain. For local anesthesia, morphine derivatives had been recommended by a Silesian oculist in the fifteenth century. Many centuries before surgeons used cocaine for local and general anesthesia, native South Americans had produced and used this narcotic. The church, however, anathematized the satanic observations of native Americans. Paracelsus probably knew about and applied ether in practice, but nobody believed or followed him in this direction. Laughing gas had been discovered in 1772 by the teacher and pastor Priestley, who also discovered oxygen in 1774. "Pneumatic" institutions were founded where it became the fashion to treat lung diseases (and later on other diseases) by inhalation of anti-inflammatory gases, as oxygen was regarded to be. A young man named Davy detected the analgesic effect of laughing gas in an experiment on his own body and published his enthusiastic report in 1800: "Nitrous oxide seems to largely eliminate physical pain which would obviously be advantageous for surgical operations"; an important hint that met with no response. However, three decades later another Englishman had an analogous experience in Shropshire: the physician and surgeon Henry Hill Hickman performed painless surgery by administering laughing gas (nitrous oxide) in animal experiments. Hickman, who at the early age of 20 was a member of the Royal College of Surgeons in London, published his results in 1824, trying in vain to call the attention of his fellow members to this effect. This is even more inconceivable as Sir Humphry Davy had just been elected president of the Royal Society , while his disciple Michael Faraday had rediscovered Paracelsus's detection of the narcotizing effect of ether. Hickman traveled to Paris in 1828, asking King Charles X to have his findings checked by the highest authority in science, the Académie Française, but with no response. Only the great Larrey supported him. Disappointed and depressed, Hickman returned to England. There was no time left for another attempt; he died in 1830, before his 30th birthday.

In the early nineteenth century, at modern parties, the effect of alcohol was intensified by inhaling narcotic gases. "Ether frolics" and "laughing gas parties" were then the latest rage in North America and Europe (Fig. 11). Obviously, this was not a

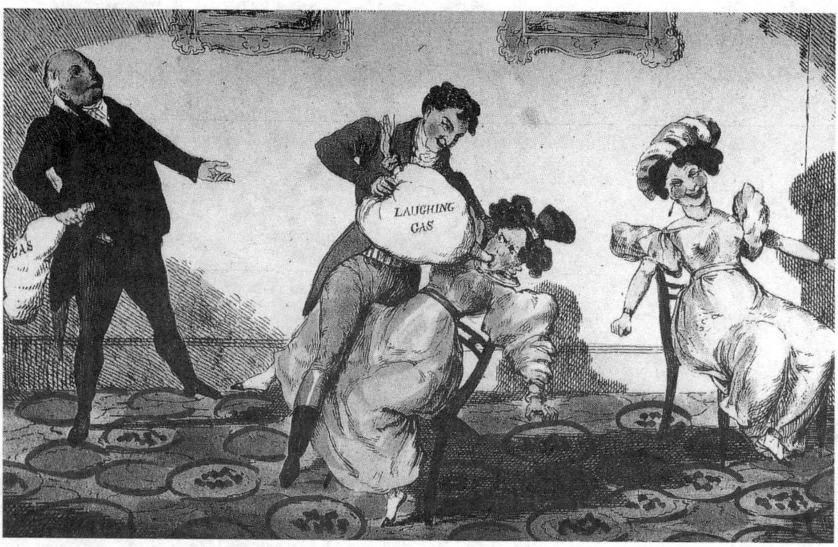

Fig. 11. Laughing gas party, London 1830

good base for the start of modern anesthesia. The famous Paris surgeon A.L.M. Valpeau (1795–1867) wrote in 1831, "The idea to prevent pain in surgery is too absurd; so it has been abandoned. Scalpel and pain will never appear separately to the patient, and we have to resign ourselves forever with their common presence."

Nevertheless, due to observations made by young Crawford William Long (1815–1878) in Jefferson, Georgia during "ether frolics", an attempt was begun to replace the brandy usually administered against pain in surgery with ether inhalations. Long used this method to painlessly remove a neck tumor in a friend of his on March 30, 1846. This was the first surgical narcosis but it only became known much later.

This contributed, ultimately, to what happened on October 16, 1846: the first public anesthesia at Massachusetts General Hospital in Boston, which opened the door for modern surgery. At Würzburg, the first ether narcosis in Germany was performed on

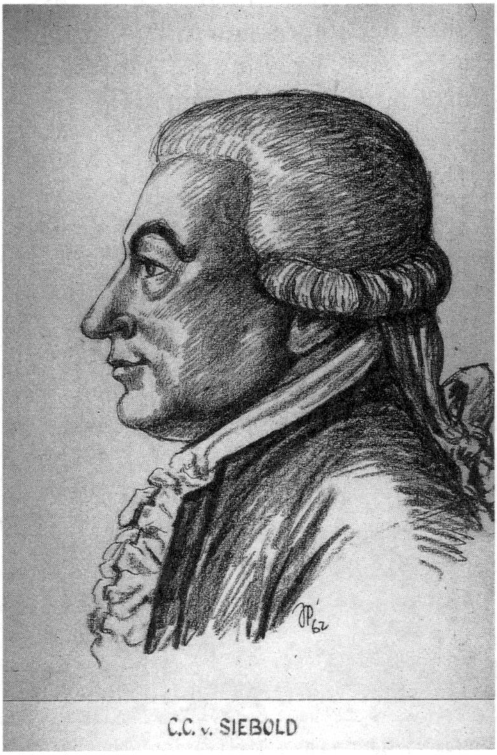

Fig. 12. C.C. von Siebold (1736–1807) "Surgeon of the south". Würzburg 1769–1807. Drawing by Ruddle: Chirurgische Universitätsklinik Würzburg

February 3, 1847 during a major operation by Cajetan von Textor. In 1816 Textor had become the successor to Elias von Siebold, son of Carl Caspar von Siebold and father of Philipp Franz von Siebold, after the basis for modern surgery had been established by the first chair-holder of anatomy, surgery and obstetrics: Carl Caspar von Siebold (1736–1807) (Fig. 12).

The most important steps in the reintroduction of anesthesia can thus be summarized as follows:

- Spain, thirteenth century: discovery of ether
- American Indians use cocaine as a drug
- Etherization by Paracelsus?
- 1772: Priestley develops laughing gas
- 1800: Davy reports on the pain-soothing effect of laughing gas
- 1824: Henry Hill Hickman reports on painless surgery in animals by means of laughing gas (nitrous oxide)
- Laughing gas parties and ether frolics
- March 30, 1846: Painless removal of a nuchal tumor by Crawford William Long (1815–1878) by means of ether inhalation
- October 16, 1846: First public and successful ether narcosis by William Thomas Green Morton (1819–1868) at Massachusetts General Hospital in Boston

When aseptic and antiseptic surgery was finally generally adopted, as a consequence of the research done by Semmelweis, Pasteur, Lister, and Koch, thus avoiding postoperative infections, two major hurdles had been cleared for modern surgery.

The time had come for the “century of surgeons” (Thorwald 1972).

References

Bochalli R (1954) Robert Koch, der Schöpfer der modernen Bakteriologie. Stuttgart

Drees A (1989) Blutiges Handwerk – Klinische Chirurgie. Zur Entwicklung der Chirurgie zwischen 1750 bis 1920 Böhnen

Fischer A (1965) Geschichte des deutschen Gesundheitswesens, 2 vol. Hildesheim

Geiger A (1983) Lorenz Heister als Begurtshelfer und gynäkologischer Chirurg. Vergleichende Untersuchung anhand der verschiedenen Auflagen seiner "Chrirugie". Züricher Medizinische Abhandlungen, Neue Reihe, Nr. 162

Gurlt E (1898) Geschichte der Chirurgie und ihrer Ausübung, 3 vol. Berlin

Haferkamp H (1989) Die Geschichte der Narkose. in: Blutiges Handwerk – Klinische Chirurgie Drees A. Bönen

Havig G (1990) Chirurgische Ausbildung im 18. Jahrhundert. Husum

Keil G (1995) Die Biographie Roger Frugardis. Lexikon des Mittelalters, vol 7, p 92

Kilian H (1980) Meister der Chirurgie und die Chirurgenschulen im gesamten deutschen Sprachraum. Stuttgart

Korff R (1975) Das Berufsethos in der Chirurgie Lorenz Heisters (1683–1758). Züricher medizinhistorische Abhandlungen, Neue Reihe Nr 107

Lyons AS, Petrocelli II, RJ (1980) Die Geschichte der Medizin im Spiegel der Kunst. DuMont

Pächter H (1955) Paracelsus. Das Urbild des Doktor Faustus. Stuttgart

Probst C (1992) Fahrende Heiler und Heilmittelhändler. Medizin von Marktplatz und Landstraße. Rosenheim

Ridder P (1993) Chirurgie und Anästhesie. Vom Handwerk zur Wissenschaft. Stuttgart

Rüster D (1986) Alte Chirurgie. Legende und Wirklichkeit. Deutscher Ärzteverlag

Rüster D (1993) Der Chirurg, ein Beruf zwischen Ruhm und Vergessen. Leipzig

Schott H (1996) Meilensteine der Medizin Harenberg. Dortmund

Skopec M (1990) Das Ringen um die Einheit von Chirurgie und Medizin am Beispiel des Wiener Josephinums. In: Harig G (ed) Chirurgische Ausbildung im 18. Jahrhundert. Husum

Sudhoff K (1936) Paracelsus. Ein deutsches Lebensbild aus den Tagen der Renaissance. Leipzig

Thiel R (1942) Männer gegen Tod und Teufel. Berlin

Thorwald J (1972) Das Jahrhundert der Chirurgen Knauer. Stuttgart

CHAPTER 3

Karl Kaspar von Siebold

G. Keil

According to the taste of his time, Karl Kaspar von Siebold was certainly an attractive person. He was almost 2 m tall, stout, well-proportioned, broad-shouldered, a good dancer, and a man who moved elegantly (Fig. 1). He overcame an injury caused by the hoof of an imperial horse so well that 5 years later he no longer limped. Karl Kaspar von Siebold was a man of the world who was able to converse in four leading European languages: German, French, Dutch and English. In addition, he knew some Spanish. He also became a member of the inheritable nobility. Archduke Carl himself, the *Salvator Germaniae*, recommended

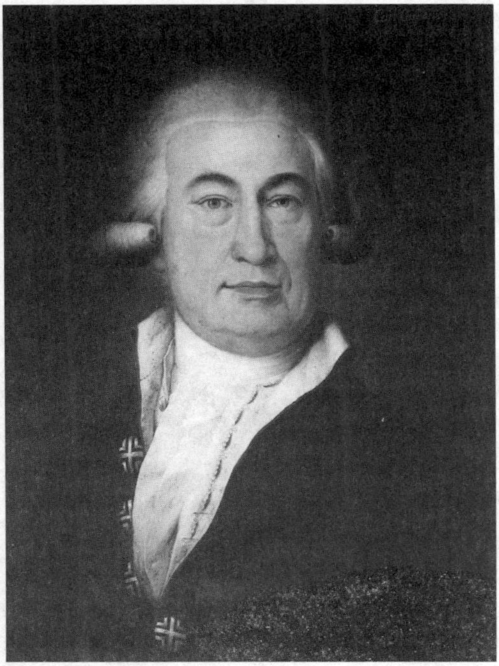

Fig. 1. Karl Kaspar von Siebold (painting by Conrad Huber, property of the Martin-von-Wagner-Museum of the University of Würzburg)

that his imperial brother should make Siebold a knight. Archduke Carl took part in the battle of Würzburg, where the victorious French army (which was involved in the French Revolution) was defeated for the first time and where the French were pushed back beyond the Rhine. The little Archduke, of whom much fun was made and whose face was marked by epilepsy, also won the battle against the revolutionaries. His victory was so overwhelming that only a large number of German politicians could ruin his success. Two thousand French soldiers died and several thousand revolutionaries were seriously injured. Sabres rattled above the city to the east of Würzburg called "Letzter Hieb". Wounded soldiers from the imperial German army could also be found. The whole city of Würzburg looked like an enormous hospital, and at the same time it seemed to be a military base. All the inhabitants of the city were busy with the injured soldiers. The seriously hurt were huddled together in the Juliusspital and in the Deutschordenshaus, an improvised hospital (Fig. 2).

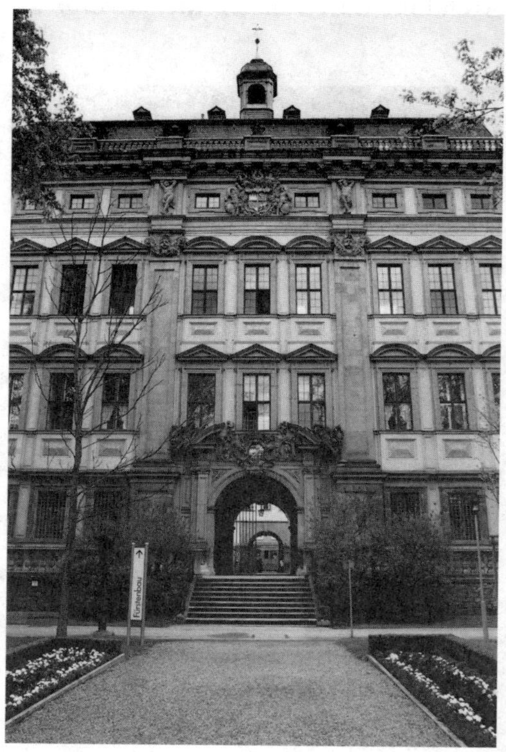

Fig. 2. The Fürstenbau (constructed by A. Pellegrini and J. Greising, baroque structure completed in 1712). During the era of K.K. von Siebold it was the seat of the administration of the Juliusspital

Karl Kaspar von Siebold, a surgeon and a professor of anatomy, surgery and gynaecology, worked among all these injured soldiers. He was a privy councillor, a physician-in-ordinary to the Archbishop and a member of various academies. Siebold showed what the world-famous surgery of Würzburg could do. He ordered his two sons who lived in Jena to come to Würzburg, where his oldest son already held a professorship. In addition, many well-educated assistant surgeons helped Siebold. They operated for 4 days and 3 nights, hardly taking a break for sleep. The field of work of the surgeons was a very wide one. They did almost everything, including resections, amputations, operations on the face and fractures of the skull. Siebold asked: "How did the hussars smash the heads of the French?" The medical doctors had not only to bandage or splint but also had to worry about dietetics and prostheses. Siebold asked: "Did you realize how many wooden legs can be seen in Würzburg? They prove how flourishing surgery is in Würzburg." Siebold provided accommodation outside Würzburg, in the surrounding villages, where he treated generals, staff-officers and troops. To the French Siebold spoke French, to the imperial dragoons he spoke German and to the Dutch auxiliary troops he spoke Dutch. All the wounded trusted him. He was nominated to become a member of the French Legion of Honour, and the Emperor offered him the big golden honour medal. Three of Siebold's students, among them the general army physicians Friedreich and Brünninghausen, were decorated with a gold medal at a public mounting of the guards.

Four years later, it was again time for the French revolutionary troops to invade Germany. The armed forces of General Augereau were in Franconia, and Würzburg was taken. The imperial dragoons, however, resisted the assault in the Marienburg fortress for 8 weeks and finally beat off Napoleon's troops successfully. In late autumn 1800, Würzburg looked like an army camp, everywhere overcrowded with wounded soldiers. Siebold and his men worked without interruption and if the 65-year-old Siebold was tired, his eyes became narrow slits. Five deep lines appeared on his face, dividing the right cheek into three parts and the left cheek into two. Thus the countenance of the surgeon seemed to be square and rough and his face seemed to be framed with bulges. However, the operating surgeon was happy and bore the superhuman burden in a good mood. "I have performed my art with pleasure", nobody "owes ... anything to me", "my reward is the consciousness of having worked for mankind", he said after 8 weeks of enormous demands and unbelievable successes. He remarked: "the war enables me to use my surgical talents, thus I was able to render the best service. I made great efforts to do so ... at the same time, the success I had hoped for appeared". Siebold added: "I may say, without showing off, that sometimes I was successful in treating (the patients) in a masterly manner." Also the commander in chief of the German troops said that "the surgeon of Würzburg ... distinguished himself by free treatment of 12 officers and 577 soldiers" in such an extraordinary way that he deserved to become a knight. Finally, on 30 September 1801, Siebold became a member of the order of knights. The Emperor noted with his own hand: "Ich will den Karl Kaspar Siebold ... in den Reichsadels-Stand ... in Gnade erheben". The Würzburg professor was very lucky and his face shone with pleasure.

The 66-year-old was proud of looking much younger than he actually was, and he liked it if people supposed that he was only in his late 40s. Siebold thought of himself as still possessing a good appearance, strength and activity. According to him, people who were healthy were young. After he became a widower in 1793, he decided to marry again. He was all the more shocked when an apoplectic seizure struck him, from which he recovered only in spring 1803. "The one who is ill is already old", he stated. "People only promise a long life to me. By the way, we are all in the hands of God. *Fiat voluntas, qua in coelo et in terra*".

It seems that Siebold had few enemies. During the 44 years of his service in Würzburg, none of his colleagues was in conflict with him. This was due to his extraordinary knowledge of human nature, combined with a Prussian sense of duty and his military precision. None of the non-commissioned surgeons, none of his assistants and none of his students ever ignored his commands. No prosector and no instrument-maker was ever tempted to disobey his orders. No midwife, no servant at the institute, no scientist ever acted contrary to his recommendations. Architects, officers and troops were obedient to him, as well as patients, and many members of his wide-spread family submitted voluntarily to his authority. Visiting scientists said: "Siebold is a warm-hearted, passionate and very clever man, but he is also a very kind and polite person." "He leads the clinical experiments of students and visiting scientists in a pedantic and exact way... He is totally a *homo ad chirurgiam natus*, and he possesses competence combined with an unshakable presence of mind."

In particular, it must be pointed out that Siebold was very charitable and hospitable. Everyone who traveled through the town was warmly welcomed in Siebold's house, which gradually developed into the forerunner of the university guesthouse. Siebold not only enjoyed having a convivial dinner and good food but he also liked to eat a lot. Although his house was always open to guests, he did not hesitate to wake them up in the middle of the night. An American who was on his way through Würzburg noted: "Tonight, immediately after I had arrived, a serious, unnatural birth took place in Siebold's surgery. He called me to attend the process. I appreciate that I didn't miss it, because I could learn a lot ... Siebold is very skilful." "I am able to form a judgement because I perform operations myself and I watch colleges operating every day."

Siebold was highly estimated as a human being and as a scientist. He was very much respected and had an extraordinary personal authority. Simple citizens, soldiers, principals, dukes and even the emperor paid tribute to him. His high social position and the fact that Siebold had become a knight of the Holy Roman Empire made him unassailable from the outside, so those who envied him had to fight him secretly.

First of all, one has to mention Joseph Heinrich Sulzbeck. He would have been totally forgotten in the history of science if he hadn't been discovered to be Siebold's opponent. It can be shown that Sulzbeck was the highest military surgeon holding the rank of a medical doctor on the general staff; thus he has to be classified as a medical official with a cabinet position. If the Archbishop attacked the professor of surgery about medical affairs, if he blamed his "disrespectful behaviour" and reproached him with having a supposed mania to dominate, if he insisted on total subordination, if he addressed Siebold gruffly: "I won't be dictated to by the laws and requirements of a surgeon, and I demand total obedience to my commands": then one recognized that Sulzbeck was the one in the background who had put obstacles in Siebold's way. He envied the surgeon all his life.

Sulzbeck referred skilfuly to the 200-year-old hospital regulations of 1618. According to these, a surgeon was regarded as a craftsman educated in the academic field and like all the other craftsmen he was under the control of the ecclesiastical head of the hospital. Sulzbeck took a kind of malicious pleasure in the idea of seeing Siebold, a professor and head of the hospital, lined up with "subordinate servants and minor characters". He liked the scene in the waiting-room where the senior person in the medical department had to wait patiently next to the domestic servant, the woman who was responsible for linen and the supervisor of the kitchen until he was allowed to be shown in. Siebold received his orders from a priest or other clergyman, and he had to listen to the instructions. The humiliation made no impression on him. He showed up in a general's uniform decorated with medals, and he was taller than all the other servants. Siebold showed off with his sword while the clergyman gave him his instructions; thus, by making fun of the short priest, he exposed the whole set-up to ridicule.

Siebold's behavior made Sulzbeck, the envious medical officer, think of revenge. It was due to Sulzbeck's activities that the priest of the institution enforced a diet for wounded patients on the director of the hospital, he restricted the visiting times and without authorization excluded postgraduate students from visits. Finally, the priest tried to stop all clinical teaching. The university hospital, with all its departments, was concerned about these restrictions. Meinolph Wilhelm, Director of the Medical Clinic, couldn't deal with the quarrel. For Siebold, however, the confrontation was a challenge. He was ready to handle it, and in the end he was the winner. On 4 October 1803 he was appointed executive medical officer of the Franconian principality, and the region of his activity was extended to Bamberg. Thus Siebold also had his way against his opponent from Bamberg, Adalbert Friedrich Marcus, who was successful in gaining the confidence of Archbishop Franz Ludwig. Adalbert Friedrich Marcus drove away all physicians-in-ordinary. He convinced the sovereign not to agree to an essential operation, and he treated Franz Ludwig with natural remedies for 16 years until he died.

Siebold was able to win against Marcus and Sulzbeck, but he was powerless against the prejudices of some esteemed ladies of high social standing. Nothing helped against their disgust and aversion. In particular, it was no help that Siebold's father became the wealthiest man and lord mayor of Nideggen; that his brother administered Comelimünster Abbey as a legal advisor and lawyer; that his brother-in-law, a pharmacist in Düren, had become very rich; that his daughter-in-law and later his granddaughter both earned doctoral degrees in obstetrics; that he himself was a doctor in the medical field as well as in philosophy; that the sovereign was benevolent towards him; that he possessed many medals; that he was an honorary member of many organizations; that the Emperor favored him, and that he was a member of the cabinet. Nor did being a nobleman help. The ladies of Würzburg regarded Siebold as one who had learned the bloody profession of a surgeon and as a stranger and parvenu whose grandfather had worked as a cook for an earl, with a father who had been a surgeon – a craftsman. From their point of view, Siebold was simply an operating surgeon, a person who shed the blood of innocent patients by cutting off legs, arms and many other parts of the body – and even worse Siebold seemed to be an anatomist and pathologist who performed autopsies, broke bones and possessed dreadful equipment. The Duchess of Bavaria was frightened to death when Siebold explained to her: "This is a coffin where the parts which are supposed to be used for demonstation ... are put in spirits". The Duke shouted: "Don't open! Don't open!", when his assistant tried to lift the cover in front of the Duchess's eyes. All the ladies agreed that Siebold was an awful man and they felt not honored but insulted if Siebold, an operating surgeon, or his wife was invited to a ball.

Siebold had to struggle hard for his professional success. Although it was not easy to make the profession of surgeon a learned one again, he tried to introduce regulations about teaching methods and examinations for Franconian surgeons. For decades, he not only demanded that surgeons should be highly respected and not regarded as minor characters, but he also kept repeating this claim. In addition, he tried hard to establish his demand legally. All these endeavors were necessary in order for success in "ennobling the profession of surgeons", Siebold stated. In other words, this was the only possibility for guaranteeing equal positions for operative and non-operative medicine. Thus Siebold's medical field became one of the "most respected medical disciplines" in the nineteenth century due to the above-mentioned development started by this famous surgeon in 1766.

Siebold's enormous success was accompanied by other important achievements, such as the installation of the first operating theater in the world; the opening of the first gynecological university hospital; the fact that the hospital of psychiatry was made independent; the introduction of no restraint for mentally ill patients (he established the policy of no restraint long before it was thought of in Paris); the elevation of midwives' education to an academic level; the introduction of compulsory insurance against illness for working craftsmen; and finally, the separation of parts of the hospital from ecclesiastical administration. It has to be stressed that the new building for a medical and theoretical institute was constructed under Siebold's management.

Siebold considered himself a conservative person, who disliked all new things and felt bound to old traditions, However, his self-estimate is not at all correct and is refuted by historically orientated analysis as well as by his effectiveness. In this paper, I don't want to take into account the numerous innovations of his doctoral students, his candidates who wanted to qualify as university lecturers, and all his other students. His innovative activities covered pathological skills, the science of performing operations, and the first description of Bell's palsy. It is much more important that Siebold and his students filled 25 professorships in Germany and abroad and that 25 of his students worked as senior medical officers. He and his sons were the first to start the German journals for surgery and gynecology. Apart from that, Siebold planned to establish a surgical academy which was intended to have its seat in Würzburg. It is important that he influenced all those who collaborated with him to an unbelievable extent. This can be proved by looking at the academic curriculum of his non-academic servants and assistants. Joseph Halberstädter, who was Siebold's secretary for many years, was nominated as professor of veterinary medicine without having any education in this field. Franz Kaspar Hesselbach, his uneducated dissection assistant, was twice offered the chair of anatomy and was appointed an honorary doctor. Thanks to Goethe, Johann Georg Heine, Siebold's instrument-maker, was made a surgical honorary doctor. Heine initiated operative orthopedics, and he and his nephew Bernhard were both awarded the Prix Montyon. This honor, comparable to the Nobel Prize, was given to the Medical Faculty of the University of Würzburg for the first and last time.

Apart from Schönlein and Virchow, Siebold was the most successful lecturer Würzburg has ever had. It was a characteristic of his strategy that he filled positions by referring to fellow students and postgraduate friends. He did not hesitate to appoint some relatives of his mother as professors and to call three of his sons to positions in Würzburg. All were excellent clinicians and proved to be good at professorial chairs in Würzburg or in other places, as can be seen for instance with the professorship for operative gynaecology in Berlin. With the grandchildren of the third generation, theoretical subjects like zoology, history of medicine and ethnology dominated. Philipp Franz von Siebold, a researcher in East Asia, was particularly famous. Only a short time ago a new museum was opened in his memory. Alexander, the great-grandson of Karl Kaspar von Siebold, became a baron in 1870 and served as a diplomat in the Far East for five decades. Highly honored by the Emperor Mutsuhito, Alexander died in 1911 while on a journey through Italy.

The University of Würzburg owes many thanks to Siebold. He called the Faculty of Medicine, which almost broke down in the middle of the century, into existence again in 1760, and from 1769 it was dominated by Siebold for almost four decades. August Gottlieb Richter, his companion on a study trip, referred to the department as the Academia Sieboldiana and thus awarded an honorary title which was in use until the nineteenth century. It was Karl Kaspar von Siebold who ensured that Würzburg would remain the site of the Julius University when he put his Bamberg opponent Marcus in the shade after Franconia had become part of Bavaria.

"*Chirurgus inter Germanos princeps*": from 1780 onward, Siebold and his companion from Paris divided the Deutsche Reich into two zones. August Gottlieb Richter dominated the northern part starting in Göttingen, while Siebold worked in the areas from Vienna to Strassburg and from Nanzig to Prague. Siebold was without dispute the "Surgeon of the South", dominating the Lower Mountains and the Alps.

CHAPTER 4

Karl Kaspar von Siebold and Anatomy in Würzburg

G. Keil

The date 8 July 1988 was a double occasion for celebration for the institution of anatomy in Würzburg: on the one hand it was the 65th birthday of one of its most highly respected members[1] ; on the other hand, a memorable event had taken place during exactly the same week 200 years earlier. On 9 July 1788, a ceremony held in Würzburg was noticed far beyond the region's frontiers[2]. What had happened? What type of occasion attracted international attention to the Prince Bishop's residence in Franconia? What made the dean of the faculty of medicine invite his sovereign for "the 9th day of next July"? What encouraged him to bluntly threaten his "High Princely Grace" that he absolutely must participate in that ceremony, not for the "glory of our uni-

[1] Johannes Lang, born in Munich on 5 July 1923, co-head of the Würzburg Institute of Anatomy from 19 July 1966 to 1 October 1991.

[2] Carl Caspar von Siebold [invitation to Franz Ludwig von Erthal, June 1788], printed by Eugen Kohlmann, Die Anatomie im juliusspitälischen Garten während des ersten Jahrhunderts ihres Bestehens (1726–1826), med. thesis, Würzburg 1960, p. 22 [cit.]; also in: Adolf Holzmann, Bernhard Mohr, Was gab es in Würzburg vor Virchow an pathologischer Anatomie und pathologisch-anatomischem Unterricht?, [med. thesis, Würzburg 1929], Virchows Arch Pathol Anat 1929, 272:531–572, here p. 539; see Hans Körner, Die Würzburger Siebold. Eine Gelehrtenfamilie des 18. und 19. Jahrhunderts, Neustadt a.d. Aisch 1967 (Quellen und Beiträge zur Geschichte der Universität Würzburg, 3), p. 49; Georg Feser, Das anatomische Institut in Würzburg 1847–1903, med. thesis, Würzburg 1978, p. 2 f.; Johannes Steudel, Die Siebolds: Ein hervorragendes Ärzte-Geschlecht aus dem Dürener Lande, Düren [1954], pp. 20 f. and 31; Mirjam Elze, Die Geschichte des anatomischen Institutes in Würzburg von 1582 bis 1848, med. thesis, Würzburg 1990, pp. 119–128.

versity and the best of our state", not for the presence of "the students and all the rest of devoted citizens", not for the dean's "ceremonial welcome address" – no! but for the celebration of something enormously "important" and "of public utility", an event that was to introduce a new "splendid epoch". This ceremony, "this glorious and interesting Grand Entrance" was not only to attract the citizens' attention "but to strike the eyes of all our good nation". What, then, was to attract patriotic interest in Würzburg from far beyond its boundaries? Which epochal event persuaded the "Father of the Country" that he absolutely had to participate? Nothing other than a new "institute", nothing other than the "ceremonial inauguration of a public school"[3], nothing other than the completion of a "new anatomic theater" in the Juliusspital gardens which had been constructed within just 1 year. However, with this "anatomic school" Würzburg's medical faculty had succeeded, for the very first time, in constructing its own building for one of its institutions. And even more: this new building gave Würzburg a leading position in Germany, next to Frankfurt and Kassel, while its anatomy equaled the standards of Paris and Leiden[4]. Moreover, the medical faculty had succeeded in developing the idea of analyzing the importance of medical schools to the state and focusing public interest, which indeed went far beyond this "theatrum anatomicum" (Fig. 1). In fact, the construction of the Juliusspital hospital started in the following year. A further result of this development was the hospital in

[3] Karl Kaspar [von] Siebold, Rede von den Vortheilen, welche der Staat durch öffentliche anatomische Lehranstalten gewinnt. Bey der feyerlichen Einweyhung des neuen anatomischen Theater gehalten, Nürnberg 1788; excerpts printed in Kohlmann (1960), pp. 18–21; also Körner (1967), pp. 50–53 and Fig. 9 (table before p. 25). The sovereign mentioned was the severely ill Prince Bishop Franz Ludwig; see Gundolf Keil (1995) *Morbus ferialis* – letzte Krankheit und Tod. Anmerkungen zur Pathographie Franz Ludwigs von Erthal, in: Baumgärtel-Fleischmann R (ed) Franz Ludwig von Erthal, Fürstbischof von Bamberg und Würzburg 1779–1795, edited by order of the Diocesan Museum of Bamberg (Veröffentlichungen des Diözesanmuseums Bamberg, 7), Bamberg, pp. 325–336.

[4] Kohlmann, see footnote 2, p. 12 f.

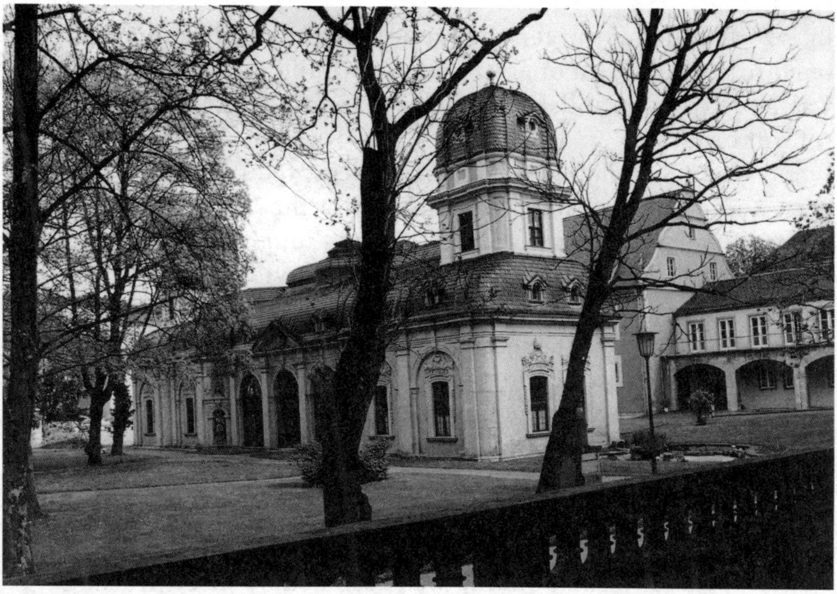

Fig. 1. The historic *theatrum anatomicum* in the gardens of the Juliusspital. Here, Albert von Koelliker (anatomist) and Robert Virchow (pathologist) carried out their scientific work

Bamberg, inaugurated in 1789; this was the prototype of a modern university clinic which was copied worldwide[5].

Why did Karl Kaspar von Siebold, dean of the medical faculty and initiator of the ceremony in 1788, start his Würzburg program of modernization with the construction of a "theatrum anatomicum"? Why did he not first install a surgical operating theater, the construction of which, 4 years later in 1802, consolidated Würzburg's glory in surgical progress?[6] History provides the answer: When Siebold was planning an institute of anatomy

[5] Dieter Jetter, Geschichte des Hospitals. I. Westdeutschland von den Anfängen bis 1850 (Sudhoffs Archiv Suppl 5), Stuttgart: Franz-Steiner-Verlag Wiesbaden 1966, pp. 63–68, 73 etc.

[6] Georg Sticker (1932) Entwicklungsgeschichte der Medizinischen Fakultät an der Alma mater Julia. In: Buchner M (ed) Aus der Vergangenheit der Universität Würzburg. Festschrift zum 350jährigen Bestehen der Universität, herausgegeben im Auftrage von Rektor und Senat. Berlin, pp. 383–799, here pp. 510–537 (without details); Steudel (1954) [see footnote 2], p. 23; Körner (1967) [see footnote 2], pp. 34, 54, 176 f., 186.

in 1776[7], academic surgery had not yet been sufficiently developed to start with an operating theater building[8], while anatomy was already an established discipline and thus a safe basis for his reform program.

When Siebold, at the age of 33, accepted the chair of "anatomy, surgery and obstetrics", anatomy at the University of Würzburg already had a long history[9]. Even though there had been no remarkable achievements during the previous 150 years, it was considered promising for academic development and substantial enough to attract the sovereign's pleasure.

In 1699, Prince Bishop Johann Philipp von Greiffenklau had renovated the fire-damaged northern wing of the Juliusspital together with the garden, which became one of the most beautiful parks of Europe. The sovereign even planned a private summer residence in it that he wished to use as a garden pavilion and a point of departure for delightful walks among fountains and flower borders[10]. The building was designed by Josef Greising with a narrow central part and broader lateral wings. At considerable expense, construction was completed after several years in 1714. However, the sovereign never used it: The Tuscan arcades, obviously, saw neither any "cheerful party" nor the intended "delights". Immediately after its completion, this incomparably elegant building must have been occupied by the anatomist Johann

---

[7] Körner (1967), p. 48, footnote 100.

[8] Efforts to this end did not begin before the 1790s; see footnote 7, p. 176; for the state of surgery around the turn of the nineteenth century, see Hans-Heinz Eulner (1970) Die Entwicklung der medizinischen Spezialfächer an den Universitäten des deutschen Sprachgebietes, Stuttgart (Studien zur Medizingeschichte des 19. Jhs, 4), pp. 295–321, particularly p. 300; Dominik Groß (1996) Berufsvererbung und soziale Herkunft der württembergischen Wundärzte im 19. Jahrhundert, Sudhoffs Arch 80:38–55; and: Die Aufhebung des Wundarztberufs im Spiegel zeitgenössischer wundärztlicher Quellen, Würzburger med.hist. Mitt. 1996; 14:459–474.

[9] Theodor Heinrich Schiebler, Zur Geschichte der Würzburger Anatomie, Würzburger med.hist. Mitt. 1983, 1:139–146; Mirjam Elze, Die Geschichte des anatomischen Institutes in Würzburg von 1582 bis 1849, med. thesis, Würzburg 1990, pp. 4–18.

[10] Kohlmann (1960) [see footnote 2], p. 3; and Elze, p. 118; Alfred Wendehorst (1981) Würzburg. Geschichte in Bilddokumenten, Munich, Fig. 68, p. 133.

Simon Bauermüller, who, at least from 1720 onward, performed his dissections and lessons there. In 1726/27, a small anatomic theater was also constructed for him[11]. This was the basis for Siebold's drastic project for a new building.

The faculty of anatomy was strong enough to attract the "high princely ... summer residence". Anatomy, as a basic university subject, was even permitted to deprive the sovereign of his hoped-for "garden delight". Anatomy had practically displaced the Prince Bishop from the Juliusspital garden, sending him to his estates in nearby Veitshöchheim. Anatomy represented a powerful lobby even without its own institution.

Anatomy is one of the foundational subjects of a university. Indeed, when Longobard and Italian physicians gathered around the year 980, anatomy was among the primary disciplines which were to form the university model during the decades to come[12]. Anatomy was considered a bastion of defensive argument against the jurists, theologians and artists who in the late Middle Ages attacked medicine by reproaching it for being too vague to be recognized as a science. Indeed, physicians were still unable to look inside the human body[13]. Anatomy was the first medical dis-

---

11 Kohlmann, p. 8; Elze, p. 119; see Alfred Wendehorst (1976) Kulturgeschichte (Das Juliusspital in Würzburg, 1), Würzburg, p. 77 f.

12 Paul Oskar Kristeller (1986) Studi sulla scuola medica salernitana, Naples (Istituto italiano per gli studi filosofici "Hippocratica civitas": Collana, 1), p. 38; George W. Corner (1927) Anatomical texts of the earlier middle ages. A study in the transmission of culture. With the revised Latin text of Anatomia Cophonis and translation of four texts, Washington (Carnegie Institution of Washington, publ. no. 364); and: On early Salernitan surgery, Bull Hist Med 1937, 5:1–32; Karl Sudhoff (1927/28) Die erste Tieranatomie von Salerno und ein neuer salernitanischer Anatomietext. Arch Gesch Math Naturw Techn 10:136–154; and: Karl Sudhoff (ed) (1928) Die vierte Salernitaner Anatomie. Sudhoffs Arch 20:33–50; Reisert (1986) [see footnote 29], pp. 43–50, with the best survey on Salernitan anatomic texts.

13 Rudolf Peitz (ed) (1978) Die 'Decem quaestiones de medicorum statu'. Ein spätmittelalterlicher Dekalog zur ärztlichen Standeskunde, Pattensen bei Hann (now Würzburg) (Würzburger medizinhistorische Forschungen, 11), pp. 12–23; Gundolf Keil and R. Peitz, 'Decem quaestiones de medicorum statu'. Beobachtungen zum Fakultätenstreit und zum mittelalterlichen Unterrichtsplan Ingolstadts, in: Der Humanismus und die oberen Fakultäten.

cipline that, on the threshold of modernity, disengaged from the ancient authorities and dared to take the leap into a new era[14]. It was also responsible for all progress in medicine during the next half millenary. No medical faculty could do without anatomy, even if it had as few as three to five chairs.

Anatomy lectures were presented at Würzburg long before a university was founded[15] in 1402 and, naturally, the subject was integrated into the standard specialties taught there. Later, the university's foundation by Johann von Egloffstein was renewed by Friedrich von Wirsberg and Julius Echter. The three professors from the medical faculty gathered for a first session in 1593. They represented the disciplines of anatomy combined with botany and theoretical surgery, which is quite a few subjects for one academic specialty[16].

Anatomy at the medieval and early modern university was a descriptive specialty for every type of structure, from humans and animals to plants. From its knowledge of the human figure,

[14] Gernot Rath (1963) Andreas Vesal im Lichte neuer Forschungen, Wiesbaden (Beiträge zur Geschichte der Wissenschaft und der Technik, 6); Eulner (1970) [see footnote 8], pp. 32–45; Loris Premuda (1957) Storia dell'iconografia anatomica, Milan; Reinhard Hildebrand (ed) (1800) Samuel Thomas Soemmerring, Vom Baue des menschlichen Körpers. Knochenlehre, as well as two papers on the osseous skull from the years 1826 and 1829 (S. Th. S. Werke, by Gunter Mann edited by Jost Benedum and Werner Friedrich Kümmel, 1), Stuttgart etc. 1997, p. 11 f.

[15] Sticker (1932) [see footnote 6], pp. 413, 416; Elze (1990) [see footnote 9], p. 3: in outlines only; Mario Lanczik (1988) Der Breslauer Psychiater Carl Wernicke. Werkanalyse und Wirkungsgeschichte, Sigmaringen (Schlesische Forschungen, 2), p. 22 f. [early history of cerebral topography at Würzburg].

[16] Elze, p. 4 f.; Sticker, pp. 437, 451 ff.

anatomy derived its task of also instructing the surgeon in his operative access to the inside of the body[17].

Anatomy is characterized by its variety of topics and methods and is also complicated by its bipolar view, which dialectically differentiates between static and functional aspects. The contrast between these different views becomes evident by looking at the earliest lecturers on anatomy, who imparted their knowledge of the structure of the human body to their students in the old town of Würzburg.

The very first anatomist in this town was probably the surgeon Ortolf von Baierland, who, in the service of the bishop or the cathedral chapter[18], lectured on general medical knowledge for surgeons. As surgical therapy was his main topic, he naturally explained some structures of the human body, but related only to organs, from a functional point of view. The manual he wrote on general medicine is a literary piece of art and easily remembered for its rough beauty; more than 200 editions and various transla-

[17] Gundolf Keil (1983) Chirurg, Chirurgie, in: Lexikon des Mittelalters, 2, col. 1845–1860; Owen H. and Sarah D. Wangensteen (1978) The rise of surgery: from empiric craft to scientific discipline, Folkstone; also see Caspar Stromayr, Practica copiosa von dem rechten Grundt deß Bruch Schnidts (Lindau 1559-67), and Jakob Ruëff, Practica in arte ophthalmica copiosa (Zürich, around 1550), [I: Faksimile, II:] Kommentar zur Faksimile-Ausgabe unter besonderer Berücksichtigung der Paracelsus-Rezeption und der Kommunikationsstruktur in chirurgischen Geheimbüchern der frühen Neuzeit, by G. Keil and Peter Proff, Darmstadt 1994; and Michael Sachs, Die Leistenbruchoperation in der Handschrift 'Practica copiosa'. Serielle Darstellung der Operationsschritte durch den Lindauer Schnittarzt Caspar Stromayr (1559), Fortschr Med 1997, 115(8):35–37, and Originalien 1:17–22; also see: Ralf Vollmuth, Traumatologie und Feldchirurgie an der Wende vom Mittelalter zur Neuzeit, dargestellt anhand der Großen Chirurgie des Walther Herman Ryff (deceased in Würzburg 1548), postdoctoral med. thesis, Würzburg 1998 (typewritten); also see Siebold's own documentation of this problem: Körner (1967) [see footnote 2], pp. 31, 34, 36, 41 etc.

[18] Hans Dünninger, Wo stand das Haus des Mag[isters] Ortolf, "arczet in Wirceburc"? Würzburger med. hist. Mitt. 1991, 9:125–133.

tions have been made, and from 1280 it was the most widely read text in Middle High German literature[19].

Completely different, however, were the specialized textbooks by Berthold Blumentrost, who was also a physician in Würzburg. His books, however, had been produced as autographs, and one copy of each exists[20]. Blumentrost, like Ortolf, had studied in Paris (not in 1240, but shortly after 1300), and he gave his scholastic lectures at Stift Haug in Würzburg. In anatomy, he lectured on procreation theory, worked on embryologic problems, and was particularly interested in the science of cerebral localization. He considered all these problems from a strictly static point of view[21]. Such a variety of subjects, methods and views obviously represented repeated grueling tests for anatomy

[19] Chapters 7–11 of his *Arzneibuch*; see G. Keil, Ortolf von Baierland (von Würzburg), in: Die deutsche Literatur des Mittelalters. Verfasserlexikon, 2, totally revised edition by Gundolf Keil, Kurt Ruh [in charge until vol. 8 (1992)], Werner Schröder, Burghart Wachinger [in charge from vol. 9 (1995)] and Franz Josef Worstbrock, Iff., Berlin and New York (1977–1978 ff), here 7 (1989), col. 67–84; Ortrun Riha, Ortolf von Baierland und seine lateinischen Quellen. Hochschulmedizin in der Volkssprache, Wiesbaden 1992 (Wissensliteratur im Mittelalter, 10); G. Keil (ed) (1993) "ein teutsch puech machen". Untersuchungen zur landessprachlichen Vermittlung medizinischen Wissens: Ortolf-Studien, 1, revised by Johannes G[ottfried] Mayer and Christian Naser, Wiesbaden (Wissensliteratur im Mittelalter, 11); Älterer deutscher 'Macer' – Ortolfs von Baierland *Arzneibuch – Herbar* des Bernhard von Breidenbach – Färber- und Malerrezepte: Die oberrheinische medizinische Sammelhandschrift des Kodex Berleburg, colored microfiche edition with introduction to the texts and description of plant illustrations and the manuscript by Werner Dressendörfer, Gundolf Keil and Wolf-Dieter Müller-Jahncke, Munich 1991 (Codices illuminati medii aevi, 13).

[20] G. Keil, Berthold Blumentrost (1978) in: Verfasserlexikon [see footnote 19], I, col. 904–906; a new edition of the *Gifttraktat* (treatise on poisons) by Konrad Goehl is expected in vol. 15 (1996/97) of the journal Würzburger med.hist. Mitt.

[21] Rüdiger Krist (1987) Berthold Blumentrosts Quaestiones disputatae circa tractatum Avicennae de generatione embryonis et librum meteorum Aristotelis. Ein Beitrag zur Wissenschaftsgeschichte des mittelalterlichen Würzburgs. I. Text, Pattensen bei Hann [now Würzburg] (Würzburger medizinhistorische Forschungen, 43).

and, as a consequence, many a derivative academic discipline split off from it. The trend towards specialization in the medical and natural sciences illustrates the variety of preclinical and clinical subdisciplines which shot up from the stem of anatomy and, in their turn, continued to ramify until the crown towered above its original stem.

Anatomy, in fact, is the academic mother of many disciplines. The extent of its ramifying subdisciplines becomes apparent from the history of the institutions in Würzburg: botany split off from anatomy in 1749 and, simultaneously, even paleontology and chemistry[22]. For all of these specialties the "professor chirurgiae et anatomiae" had been responsible; he had even directed the development of the "laborationes chymicae" in the gardens of the Juliusspital[23]; he had initiated the fossil collection of Franconian shell-limestone; following his instructions, greenhouses had been built for exotic plants, and he succeeded in cultivating the 3-m high giant cactus *Cereus spinosa* with blossoms – a most remarkable event that attracted scientists and the curious from far and near in 1717[24]. The chairs of botany and chemistry with direct roots in anatomy had been established and integrated into the medical faculty in 1749[25]; the chair of history of the natural sciences, however, was not established until 1792, and it was integrated into the philosophy faculty[26]. No wonder, therefore, that

[22] Sticker (1932) [see footnote 6], pp. 476–479, 491 ff., 495, 497–500; Uwe Buschbom (1982) Die Entwicklung des Würzburger Botanischen Gartens, in: Baumgart P (ed) Vierhundert Jahre Universität Würzburg. Eine Festschrift, herausgegeben im Auftrag der Bayerischen Julius-Maximilians-Universität, Neustadt a. d. Aisch (Quellen und Beiträge zur Geschichte der Universität Würzburg, 6), pp. 567–600; Wilhelm Simonis, Zur Entwicklung der Würzburger Botanik, in: ib., pp. 601–636, here p. 603: "Professor quartus der Anatomie und Botanik [Johann Barthel] Adam Beringer", p. 607.

[23] Sticker, loc. cit., p. 481; Klaus Koschel, Die Entwicklung und Differenzierung des Faches Chemie an der Universität Würzburg, in: Baumgart, Festschrift (1982) [see footnote 22], pp. 703–750, here p. 707.

[24] Sticker, loc. cit., pp. 483–487; Hans Franke, Die Würzburger Lügensteine, Würzburg 1991, p. 17; Wendehorst (1976) [see footnote 11], p. 73.

[25] Sticker, loc. cit., p. 498 f.

[26] Sticker, loc. cit., p. 493; Siegfried Matthes, Zur historischen Entwicklung des Faches Mineralogie an der Universität Würzburg, in: Baumgart, Festschrift (1982) [see footnote 22], pp. 683–702, here p. 684.

the anatomist Karl Kaspar Siebold continued to be responsible for geologic sciences and, behind the "locked glass doors" of his "beautiful cabinets" in his 200-year-old institute of anatomy, still preserved the "rarities of nature"[27]. And what about the later history of those early scions of anatomy in Würzburg? In 1803, a second chair of chemistry was founded, which signaled its exodus to the philosophy faculty but also initiated the beginning of the exodus of pharmacy; both branches have since become autonomous specialties[28]; the same is true for the chairs merged into the geologic sciences.

In 1803, anatomy even abandoned its clinical operative branches: surgery installed an ultra-modern operating theater, and the gynecologic hospital was inaugurated in 1805. This was the signal for their further autonomy from anatomy; these branches were strong enough to follow their own academic path. However, close relationships to the mother specialty were never abandoned and up to the present day anatomy is for many a surgical specialty.

---

[27] Sticker, loc. cit., p. 518; Steudel (1954) [see footnote 2], pp. 20–22; Kohlmann (1960) [see footnote 2], p. 14 [cit.]; Körner (1967) [see footnote 2], pp. 31 f., 49 f., 65 f., 72; Wendehorst (1976) [see footnote 10], pp. 77–81; also see Theodor Heinrich Schiebler, Anatomie in Würzburg (von 1593 bis zur Gegenwart), in: Baumgart, Festschrift (1982) [see footnote 22], pp. 985–1004, here pp. 988–990; Elze (1990) [see footnote 9], pp. 50, 57 f.

[28] Sticker, loc. cit., pp. 542 f., 560; Koschel (1982) [see footnote 23], pp. 713–717 and Fig. 57 f. It refers to the academic specialties established in 1974/75, i.e., no. 8: chemistry and pharmacy (natural sciences II), and no. 7: biology (natural sciences I) with "botanics and pharmakognosis" = "botanics and pharmaceutic biology". For geosciences see Matthes (1982) [see footnote 26] and Helmut Jäger, Die Geographie an der Universität Würzburg 1593–1981, in: Baumgart, Festschrift (1982) [see footnote 22], pp. 637–664; Walter Schnitzer and Herbert Voßmerbäumer, Zur Geschichte von Geologie-Paläontologie, in: ib., pp. 665–682. For surgery and gynecology and their separation from anatomy see Sticker, loc. cit., pp. 524–526; Körner (1967) [see footnote 2], p. 175 f.; Steudel (1954) [see footnote 2], p. 36; also see Ernst Kern, Zur Geschichte der Chirurgie an der Universität Würzburg, in: Baumgart, Festschrift (1982) [see footnote 22], pp. 827–840, here p. 831

Academic anatomy in the eleventh century was veterinary anatomy[29], and so it continued even when human bodies were admitted for dissection.

In Würzburg, the regulations of 1610 particularly order the anatomist not to dissect human bodies alone, but also to practice with "corpora beluina"[30]. So, obviously, anatomy in Würzburg in the early nineteenth century integrated the subspecialties of physiology, anthropotomy and zootomy[31]. Its biogenetic research attracted international attention[32], and it became the successor institution to the dissolved academy of veterinary medicine[33]: in 1825, the anatomist Heusinger established an institute of zootomy in the veterinary medicine building, which gave an essential impetus to zoology, which had its own chair from 1830 onward and, for the time being, was the natural domain of anatomists in Würzburg. In 1870, the institute of anatomy formed its own institute of zootomy in succession to that founded by Heusinger[34].

[29] The first anatomic lectures during the high Middle Ages grew out of the 'Anatomia porci [Pseudo-]Cophonis', with pig cadavers used for dissections; see previous footnote 12 and the survey on Salernitan anatomic texts by Robert Reisert (1986) Der siebenkammerige Uterus. Studien zur mittelalterlichen Wirkungsgeschichte und Entfaltung eines embryologischen Gebärmuttermodells, Pattensen bei Hann [now Würzburg] (Würzburger medizinhistorische Forschungen, 39).

[30] Sticker (1932) [see footnote 6], pp. 477, 498.

[31] Sticker, loc. cit., pp. 552 ff., 560, 566, 604; Elze (1990) [see footnote 9], pp. 71–115; G. Keil (1998) Physiologie in Würzburg. Mit Anmerkungen zum Prioritätsanspruch Breslaus, in: Herde P, Schindling A (eds) Universität Würzburg und Wissenschaft in der Neuzeit. Beiträge zur Bildungsgeschichte. Fschr. Peter Baumgart (Quellen und Forschungen zur Geschichte des Bistums und Hochstifts Würzburg, 53), Würzburg, pp 191–208.

[32] Sticker, loc. cit., p. 554 ff.

[33] The Thierarzneyschule (veterinary school) of Würzburg had been inaugurated in 1793 (Sticker, loc. cit., p. 532), 30 years after that of Lyon, and ranks among the world's oldest veterinary schools; it was closed in 1869 because of long-lasting neglect by the authorities; see Angela von den Driesch (1989) Geschichte der Tiermedizin: 5000 Jahre Tierheilkunde, Munich, p. 167, Table 6.

In fact, anatomy in Würzburg is the mother discipline of clinical-theoretical and preclinical specialties: in 1845, the chair of pathology was established in the institute of anatomy[35], in 1865 that of physiology[36]. Both foundations reveal Rinecker's influence[37]. He was an inspired university strategist who developed ideas to counter regional politics and prevent the University of Würzburg from shrinking during the nineteenth century. He continuously created new specialties[38]; from 1840 onward, he purposely supported microscopy and physiology; in 1842, he also

[34] Sticker, loc. cit., pp. 597, 604, 668; Theodor Heinrich Schiebler (1995) Rudolf Albert von Koelliker (1817–1905), Anatom, in: Baumgart P, Süß PA (eds) Lebensbilder bedeutender Würzburger Professoren, Neustadt a. d. Aisch (Quellen und Beiträge zur Geschichte der Universität Würzburg, 8), pp. 61–90: "zootomisches Institut"; Wolfgang Speckner (1982) Carl Friedrich von Heusinger: Sein Leben und sein Wirken in Würzburg, med. thesis, Würzburg, pp. 53–69: "Zootomisches Institut"; Gerhard Krause and Martin Lindauer (1982) Die Zoologie in Würzburg vom Naturalien-Kabinett des Pater Bonavita Blank bis zur Theorie der Chromosomenindividualität von Theodor Boveri, in: Baumgart, Festschrift [see footnote 22], pp. 629–636, here p. 631: "Zoologisch-zootomisches Institut"; G. Keil, Physiologie in Würzburg [see footnote 31], pp. 203–206.

[35] Sticker, loc. cit., p. 621 f.; Adolf Holzmann (1929) Bernhard Mohr, Was gab es vor Virchow an pathologischer Anatomie und pathologisch-anatomischem Unterricht? (med. thesis, Würzburg 1928) Virchows Arch Pathol Anat 272:531–572, here pp. 564–566; Ernst Werner Kohl (1976) Virchow in Würzburg, Pattensen bei Hann [now Würzburg] (Würzburger medizinhistorische Forschungen, 6), p. 11 f.; Gundolf Keil (1980) Zur Überlieferung von Virchows Würzburger Sektionsprotokollen, Sudhoffs Arch 64:287–297, here pp. 287, 288: Bernhard Mohrs 'Zuwachs-Catalog' 1843–1848.

[36] Alexander Zuber (1989) Veratrin. Zur Entstehungs- und Wirkungsgeschichte des Bezold-Jarisch-Reflexes. With a [synoptically translated] facsimile of the Breslavian thesis by Ludwig Hirt, Pattensen near Hannover [now Würzburg] (Würzburger medizinhistorische Forschungen, 48), pp. 65–70; G. Keil, Physiologie in Würzburg [see footnote 31], pp. 205f.

[37] Gundolf Keil (1995) Franz von Rinecker (1811–1883), Mediziner, in: Baumgart, Lebensbilder [see footnote 24], pp. 20–59.

[38] Keil (1995), pp. 31–44, 52 f.; Christiane Scherg-Zeisner (1973) Die ärztliche Ausbildung an der königlich-bayerischen Julius-Maximilians-Universität 1814–1872, med. thesis, Würzburg.

initiated the course of microscopy that later was to become so famous in Würzburg; finally, he was the one who, particularly for microscopy, offered the chair to Kölliker (1847)[39] and to Virchow (1849)[40]. Microscopic anatomy and pathology represented the tools by which Rinecker prevented the University of Würzburg from shrinking; indeed, under his auspices, the number of medical students in Würzburg was the highest among German medical faculties for several decades[41].

Anatomists and pathologists of the University of Würzburg gained an international reputation due to the work of Rinecker's assistant Leydig[42] and the chairs he offered to Kölliker and Virchow, both from the school of Müller[43]. The same is true for some of Kölliker's successors in anatomy at Würzburg. Although several anatomic branches such as zoology became autonomous faculties, and although physiology itself subdivided into physiologic chemistry[44] and, during the 1870s, had a significant impact on pharmacology[45], the original faculty was still a complex one.

[39] Keil (1995) [see footnote 37], pp. 53–55; Keil (1998) [see footnote 31], pp. 202–204; Schiebler (1995), pp. 62–64; Rolf Pfeffer (1982) Prof. Franz von Rinecker 1811–1883, med. thesis, Würzburg, p. 36, according to Feser (1978), p. 38.

[40] Kohl (1976) [see footnote 35], pp. 15–24.

[41] Scherg-Zeisner (1973) [see footnote 38], p. 108.

[42] Franz von Leydig was particularly important in the development of the new medical paradigm cellular pathology; see Feser (1978) [see footnote 2], pp. 60 f., 254–257; Keil (1995) [see footnote 37], p. 50; Schiebler (1982) [see footnote 27], p. 995 f.; François Duchesneau, Genèse de la théorie cellulaire, Montreal and Paris 1987 (Collection 'Analytiques', 1), pp. 258, 287 footnote 1, 341 f.

[43] As per Hans Müller's student Albert Kölliker [Rudolf Albert von Koelliker after his ennoblement in 1897], see Schiebler, loc. cit., p. 61 f., according to Feser (1978), p. 36.

[44] Personal chair for Dankwart Ackermann in Würzburg, 1929; see Eulner (1970) [see footnote 8], p. 670; Holger Münzel (1991) Max von Frey. Leben und Wirken unter besonderer Berücksichtigung seiner sinnesphysiologischen Forschung, Würzburg (Würzburger medizinhistorische Forschungen, 53), p. 175.

[45] Dietrich Henschler (1982) Zur Entwicklung der Pharmakologie und Toxikologie, in: Baumgart, Festschrift [see footnote 22], pp. 1031–1046, here p. 1033.

After every clinical and functional subdiscipline had split off, anatomy still consisted of a wide variety of subjects, and it also developed new methods which reanimated its relationship with the operative disciplines as well as the traditional dialectic exchange on static and functional viewpoints. Hans Petersen[46] was a twentieth-century expert in the original professional tradition. In 1925, he began to add dynamic aspects, mastering both natural and philosophical sciences, so it is not surprising that, from 1932 onward, he himself lectured on the history of medical science, thus binding this discipline to the institute of anatomy for the following 20 years[47], until an institute for the history of medicine was founded in the building of the institute of anatomy. In 1952, anatomy had split off from the faculty of medical history, traditionally chaired by an anatomist[48]. This was the last historic step in the development of the Institute of Anatomy in Würzburg.

Karl Kaspar von Siebold founded the Institute of Anatomy in Würzburg on 8 July 1788; the history of anatomy, however, reaches back more than 700 years, marked by continuity and changes. Let us compare present and past by means of the same problem: two different illustrations of access to the brain that have their origin 700 m away in local distance and 700 years

---

[46] Schiebler (1982) [see footnote 27], p. 999, according to: Hans-Georg Münch (1978) Das Anatomische Institut in Würzburg von 1925–1966, med. thesis, Würzburg, pp. 17–19; also see p. 22.

[47] When Hans Petersen retired in 1940, the new head of the institute, Curt Elze, lectured regularly on medical history from the winter term of 1940/41 until the summer term of 1951 (Münch, loc. cit., p. 22). For the winter term of 1951/52, he then entrusted the continuation of his well-frequented and most popular lectures on medical history to the care of the anatomist and art historian, Robert Herrlinger, who had moved from Posen to Würzburg; see Michael Quick (1987) Sticker versus Herrlinger. Zur Benennungsmotivation des Würzburger medizinhistorischen Instituts, Würzburger med. hist. Mitt. 1987, 5:13–40; the same, Bibliographie Robert Herrlinger (1914–1968): Korrekturen, Ergänzungen und Kommentar zu den Vorarbeiten Edith Feiners, ib. 8 (1990), pp. 307–324.

[48] Who (e.g., Herrlinger) continued as such and whose anatomic pocket atlas has been in print up to the present day; Quick ([1990], p. 314) follows this ‘pocket book’ until its 17th edition.

away in time. The first is this town's oldest anatomic graphic representation[49], made by the physician Berthold Blumentrost[50]. He moved from Upper Germany to Würzburg for a position as a canon and has the same origins as his recent successor, whose anniversary was celebrated in 1988 and who created a dissection model from the same perspective, showing the elegance of modern manual art of dissection.

[49] Gundolf Keil (1990) Ortolfs chirurgischer Traktat und das Aufkommen der medizinischen Demonstrationszeichnung, in: Harms W (ed) Text und Bild, Bild und Text. DFG-Symposion 1988, Stuttgart (Germanistische Symposien, Berichtsband 11), pp. 117, 120 f., 134, 137–149, 216–221, 237 f., Figs. 41–52; also: Erltraut Auer and Bernhard Schnell (eds) Der 'Wundenmann'. Ein traumatologisches Schema in der Tradition der 'Wundarznei' des Ortolf von Baierland, in: Keil, "ein teutsch puech machen" (1993) [see footnote 19], pp. 349–401; also see Hilde-Marie Groß, Illustrationen in medizinischen Sammelhandschriften. Eine Auswahl anhand von Kodizes der Überlieferungs- und Wirkungsgeschichte des 'Arzneibuchs' Ortolfs von Baierland, in: ib. pp. 172–348.

[50] According to the illustration by Krist (1987) [see footnote 21], front view; also see the reproduction by Mario [Horst] Lanczik (1988) Der Breslauer Psychiater Carl Wernicke: Werkanalyse und Wirkungsgeschichte als Beitrag zur Medizingeschichte Schlesiens, Sigmaringen (Schlesische Forschungen, 2), pp. 21–24: "Die Lokalisationstheorien im Mittelalter".

CHAPTER 5

Philipp Franz von Siebold's Youth in Würzburg (1796–1820)

W. Dettelbacher

Philipp Franz Balthasar Siebold (Fig. 1) was born in Würzburg on 17 February 1796 and baptized the same day in the bishop's cathedral[1].

Why such a hurry? At that time, many babies risked not surviving for long, such as one of Siebold's elder brothers who died at the age of 6, and a younger sister who lived only 31 days. Baptism, however, redeemed infants from original sin and gave access to the Catholic Church. Two clergymen stood as godfathers: Philipp Balthasar Balbus of Neumünster church and Dr. Franz Lotz, eldest brother of the child's mother.

[1] The baptismal register of Würzburg high cathedral.

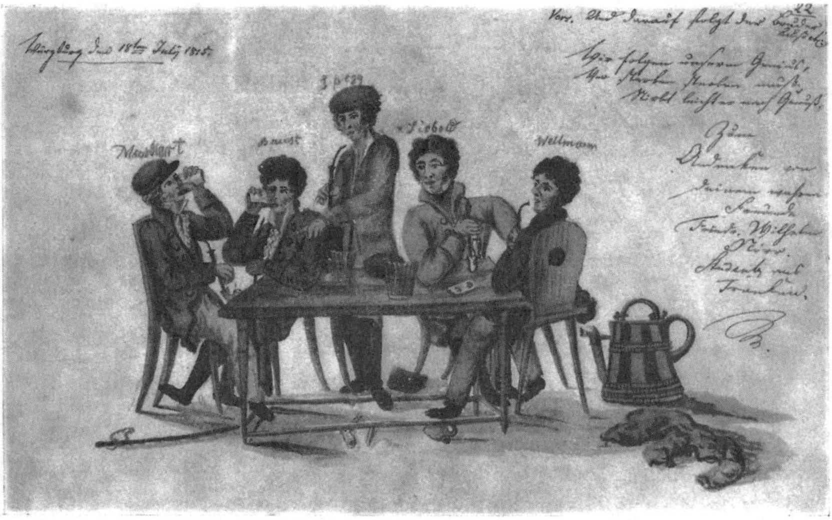

Fig. 1. Philipp Franz von Siebold (*second from right*) with his fellow students

Christoph Siebold, the father, was 29 years old. He had accepted a chair 13 months earlier and was professor of medicine and second physician at the country's most important hospital, the Julius hospital. In January 1795 he had married Appolonia Lotz, 1 year younger than himself and second daughter of Stephan Lotz, who succeeded to his father's office as a university administrator of the monastic estate of Mariaburghausen, near Haßfurt on the River Main. Prince Bishop Julius Echter had secularized the estate and donated it, with its large forest, to the university he had founded in 1582. From his youth Christoph Siebold, like his three younger brothers, was destined to become a physician and often visited the hospital where his father was head surgeon. During the investigation of a problem with a ghost[2] the 17-year-old boy was the only one who showed good sense. His father Carl Caspar took care of his education by engaging additional private teachers while he attended secondary school. The father[3] himself was born at Nideggen/Eifel in 1736, the son of a surgeon and town-councillor. His path to university had been much more difficult. After grammar school at Nideggen and secondary school at Düren, he enrolled at the University of Cologne at the age of 16 but interrupted his studies when his mother became seriously ill. His father therefore taught him the skills of a surgeon. In 1757, during the third Silesian War, he decided to enroll as a subsurgeon in the French army, as the best surgeons of the time were to be found there. The hospitals not only offered wound healing but also gave instruction on anatomy and dissection.

In winter 1759/60, 8000 men from electoral Saxon regiments were quartered in the Prince Bishop's state of Würzburg and the French headquarters sent several skilled surgeons to undertake their care. One of these was Carl Caspar Siebold. He planned to expand his knowledge and experience at the Juliusspital, a large hospital with a home for the aged and wards for epi-

[2] Arthur Bechtold (1940) Das Gespenst in der Juliusspitalmühle (The mill ghost of Juliusspital). In: Arthur Bechtold (ed) Aus dem alten Würzburg. Würzburg, p. 209f

[3] Hans Körner (1967) Carl Caspar von Siebold. In: Die Würzburger Siebold. Eine Gelehrtenfamilie des 18. und 19. Jahrhunderts [An 18th and 19th century family of scholars]. Neustadt/Aisch, pp. 465–545

leptics and mental diseases as well as for sick craftsmen. He became acquainted with the operating surgeon Christoph Stang, who demonstrated anatomy and was in charge of the midwives. When Siebold was offered the position of senior journeyman he left the army and in 1760 enrolled at the university. However, he and eight other medical students had to urge the Prince Bishop, who was rector of the university, to remind the five professors of their duty to give lectures. When he obtained first-class honors for his examination in 1763, Prince Bishop Adam Friedrich von Seinsheim (ruling 1755–79) sent him to Paris, Rouen, London, and Leiden for further studies for a total period of 30 months. On his return he became surgeon-in-ordinary to the Prince Bishop, professor of medicine and head surgeon of the Juliusspital. This made him one of the three directors of the Juliusspital, together with the hospital's clergyman and its administrator. First he developed anatomy and established a modern anatomic "theater" in the hospital garden's pavilion. In his position as public head of the midwives he was responsible for adequate instruction for them and for students of obstetrics. As a surgeon he combined theory and practice, which was unusual for that time. During operations he offered access to students from home and abroad, even to army-surgeons and city-barbers.

In addition to his father's practical instructions Christoph Siebold[4] frequented the universities of Altdorf and Göttingen, Göttingen was the most modern university of that time and in 1789, he took his doctor's degree there on obstetric cushions and chairs. He practiced for a year and in 1790 became associate professor of general medicine, dietetics, and obstetrics. He succeeded in installing a temporary maternity hospital in the Freihaus at Innerer Graben 18, where he gave practical lectures assisted by the city midwife. Like his father, he had leave for studies in Vienna and Pavia. In the summer term he obtained the chair of physiology.

In autumn 1796, the Siebold family had to undergo a crucial test of efficiency. During the battle near Würzburg on 3 September, Archduke Karl defeated the French general Jourdan. For 3 long days and nights, father and son and the three younger

[4] See note 3, pp. 546–560.

sons who had been called home from their studies in Jena operated with the local surgeons to save 589 Austrian and 200 French soldiers from tetanus and gangrene. For this unique act of rescue Carl Caspar, with his legitimate male and female heirs, was raised to the nobility of the Empire in 1801[5]. Christoph Siebold was unable to enjoy this honor. Exhausted by his consulting duties in the town, by numerous lectures and by preparations for planned manuscripts, he died from pulmonary phthisis in 1798. The former family solidarity makes us assume that his widow and her son aged 23 months found some support from her father-in-law and her brothers-in-law. She had to wait a long time for a widow's pension and repeatedly sue the university and the Juliusspital. Grandfather Carl Caspar, now more than 60 years old, still fulfilled many offices and duties. He regularly invited "touring fellows in art" to his house (Theaterstraße 18) and he used to assemble his family in the evenings. He was pleasant company and loved a good glass of wine. He was accompanied by his daughter Clara and his son Elias, who was then editor of the magazine *Lucina* (intended to improve the art of obstetrics). (His brother Barthel edited the *Neue Würzburger gelehrte Anzeigen* from 1799 to 1802, as well as *Chiron*, a periodical for surgeons, from 1805 to 1813.)

The grandfather was a good violinist and appointed musical instructors for his sons and grandsons. As he died in 1807, he was unable to enjoy listening to his son Elias as a successful concert singer or his grandson Eduard as a pianist at the age of nine. The latter mentioned that he received instruction from the city drummer in order to train his wrists.

We do not know of any public performance by Philipp Franz, but he had a piano with him in Nagasaki that still existed 140 years later in 1965. He also mastered transcription and published Japanese melodies entitled *Japanische Weisen* in Leiden in 1836.

After his father's death, Philipp Franz was placed under the care of a guardian, Dr. Franz Lotz, one of his godfathers. According to the opinion of that time, the guardian was responsible not only for his ward's spiritual salvation but also for his psychological and physical welfare.

---

[5] See note 3, pp. 510–513.

Once Dr. Lotz's theological studies had been completed, he became chaplain and private tutor (instructor) to the noble family of Freiherren von Pölnitz; then, in 1797, he was put in charge of the vicarage of Gänheim, near the Prince Bishop's summer castle of Werneck. In 1808, he was appointed parson of Heidingsfeld, a small town on the Main river near Würzburg. He now called on his sister Appolonia to act as housekeeper of his parsonage.

At the same time, he prepared his nephew for the admittance examination to the grammar school that had existed since 1561. The boy had already received instruction in mathematics and geography at Gänheim. We read in part XII of Dr. Lotz's last will[6]:"I wish my above mentioned nephew Dr. Ph. Fr. Knight of Siebold, my former pupil and my pride, to receive in my memory a portrait of mine with a big and excellently beautiful globo terrestri. I enclose those first instructions of mathematic geography which you, my dearest nephew, received in abstract from me when you were a boy of eight years." Dr. Lotz probably did not bequeath all his library to Philipp Franz, as he already possessed his own huge library at Leiden.

Dr. Lotz's main intention was to make a "foundation of a municipal library of public benefit" looked after by the parson in charge. Eleven theological volumes had been given to a clergyman, but there were still plenty of books on agriculture, bee-keeping, veterinary knowledge, geography, and ethnology.

In November 1810, Philipp Franz entered the grammar school at Würzburg, which was based on three classes in Latin school and which led to university entrance with three classes in grammar and two in rhetoric. Most important was Latin, with 5 hours reserved for the classics in the upper form.

When his cousin Eduard, due to his father's call to Berlin, entered the local grammar school, Graues Kloster (grey convent), his knowledge of Latin was far superior to that of his school fellows, but in history and mathematics he could not compete at all. In French he needed private assistance.

The same was true for Philipp Franz, as French lessons were elective and took place only once a week. In September 1814, he won a prize for doing well in French and religion[7]. He wrote

[6] This last will is filed in the bishop's archives.

his most important manuscripts in Latin, the scholars' language. This language became obsolete, however, when Alexander von Humboldt wrote his 30-volume report on South and Middle America in French.

When Philipp Franz matriculated at the university faculty of medicine in November 1815, there was no longer a Siebold lecturing. His uncle Barthel, professor of surgery and head surgeon of Juliusspital, died in January 1814 from epidemic typhus acquired in infirmaries. His uncle Elias had a chair as professor of obstetrics and was senior officer of health in Berlin, from 1816. The student matriculated in chemistry. The practical course took place in a separate experimental institution outside the town, for fear of explosions. Botany was taught by Professor Ambrosius Rau, who in 1822 suggested that Philipp Franz should be accepted as a member of the imperial Leopoldinische-Carolinische Akademie der Naturforscher (academy of natural scientists)[8].

It was a lucky chance for him that Professor Ignaz Döllinger, the friend of his father's youth, admitted him to live in his house in the Rückermain building (Karmelitenstr. 20) for a year in the winter term of 1816. The large first floor sheltered not only Döllinger's large family but also his collections and study rooms as well as two rooms reserved for students able to help the professor in his projects. In exchange, Döllinger allowed them to profit from his collections and generously shared the results of his research with them. As the founder of comparative anatomy, Döllinger had just completed a spectacular project concerning "the development of the chicken in its egg." His disciple Karl Ernst von Baer had convinced a compatriot named Heinrich Christian Pander, a banker's son from Riga, to finance these studies and to have the manuscript[9] illustrated with numerous drawings by the graphic artist d'Alton. Philipp Franz learnt there neat dissection

[7] Annual report on all youngsters studying at the Würzburg royal grammar school, with nomination of those distinguished for their performance on 17 September. p. 6 (the only known copy of the Corps Moenania archives).

[8] See note 3: Philipp Franz von Siebold, pp. 804–939, here: p. 808.

[9] Heinrich Christian Pander (1819) Historia metamorphoseos quam ovum incubatum prioribus quinque diebus ubit. Wirceburgi.

and the coloring and precise design of dissections. Later, in Japan, he profited from this instruction.

Döllinger loved to organize excursions where members of every faculty were welcome. He explored the forests of Guttenberg and Gramschatz and the parks of the castles of Veitshöchheim and Werneck, but he preferred to go to Sickershausen near Kitzingen, where since 1802 the botanist Nees van Esenbeck had a famous collection of native birds, insects and plants. In 1818, he accepted an invitation to take the chair of professor of botany in Bonn.

Philipp Franz, who grew up in a parsonage with no brothers or sisters, was introduced by his schoolfellow Spegg to the students' association Moenania (since 1820 called the Corps Moenania) which he joined in 1816[10]. According to tradition, he fought more than 30 duels, which made him a respected person among his fellow students. He answered an apparently critical letter from his uncle Elias with the remark: "I am approaching my profession day by day; I plan to work hard next summer. My uncle (Dr. Lotz) will have informed you that my professors are satisfied with my work. One learns by daily experience and I do not intend just to whirl around in life"[11]

In September 1820, Philipp Franz passed the medical examination with the vote of "excellent". On 9 October he underwent the public "disputation" which, at that time, was the major route to advancement. The disputation was presided over by Professor Döllinger and Philipp Franz had to defend, in Latin, 35 theses and three terms of study[12] against Professor Textor and Professor Ruland. As soon as he passed this procedure, he was promoted by the dean of the medical faculty and was entitled to be a doctor of medicine, surgery, and obstetrics. Thus he fulfilled the promise given to his uncle Elias: "I will close with the repeated prom-

[10] Karl Fröhlich (1899) Chronik des Corps Moenania in Würzburg vom Tage seiner Gründung bis auf die Gegenwart [Chronicles of the Corps Moenania at Würzburg from the day of its foundation until the present] 1814–1898. Würzburg, pp. 21f.

[11] Letter of 16 July 1818. Original in the archives of Brandenstein-Zeppelin, castle of Brandenstein.

[12] Staatsarchiv Würzburg, Leihgabe of Historischer Verein [historical association], Ms. 9.74, collection Köl, S-Z.

ise that I will honor the name of Siebold and, if Heaven agrees, maintain it in the memory of Würzburg."

CHAPTER 6

Siebold as a Surgeon, Physician and Medical Teacher in Japan

S. Hiki, Y. Hiki

Introduction

Philipp Franz von Siebold (1796–1866), a German physician, landed at Nagasaki in August 1823 (Fig. 1) as a physician working in a Dutch settlement. Under the national seclusion policy of the Tokugawa Shogunate, Japan's doors were closed to the West from the seventeenth to the nineteenth centuries, and Japan had no trade relations with any countries except China and Holland; entry into the country was therefore denied to all Europeans apart from the Dutch. Siebold entered Japan as a Dutchman, despite his German accent.

Siebold was employed by the East India Company and was sent to Japan as a medical doctor working for a Dutch factory. In Nagasaki, he treated not only Dutch but also Japanese patients. Eventually, his fame as a surgeon, medical scholar and educator spread not only in Nagasaki but throughout the country. Siebold performed great services in establishing western medicine in Japan.

Medical Treatment in Japan Before the Arrival of Siebold

In Japan, medical treatment before the introduction of western medicine was based on Chinese medicine. Specialists in gynecology and ophthalmology had already appeared in Japan in the fourteenth century, and Chinese medicine was systematized by Dousan Manase in the sixteenth century. However, the field of surgery was still rudimentary. Most Japanese medicine in those days consisted of internal medicine, including the use of Chinese remedies. Early European medicine was eventually introduced to

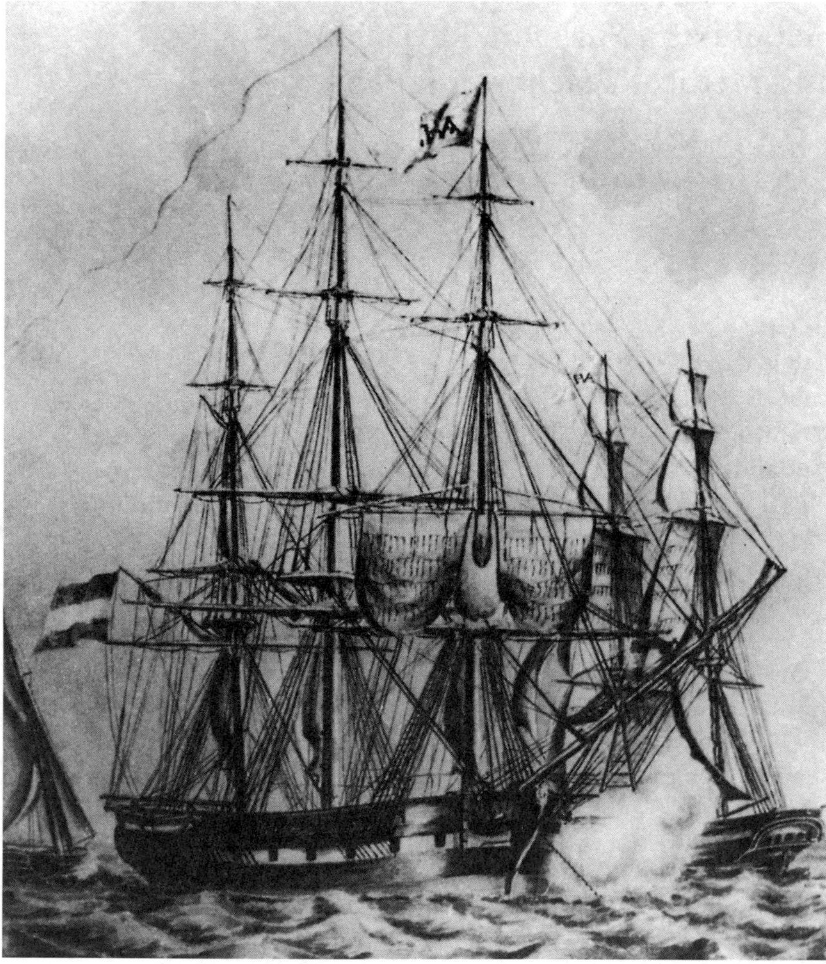

Fig. 1. The Dutch frigate Jongen Adriane in which Siebold embarked for Java

Japan by Portuguese and Spanish traders and missionaries, including Francisco Xavier at the beginning of the seventeenth century, and surgical treatment was then performed in Nagasaki for the first time. In those days, France was a leading nation in the field of medicine, and Ambroise Paré had already written many books on surgery. Some of his books were translated into Dutch and were later brought to Japan in 1706 [1].

Thus western medicine was introduced to Nagasaki, the only city in Japan open to Europe at that time, via Holland, and many young Japanese doctors were attracted to Nagasaki to study the new Dutch medicine.

Even before Siebold's day, Germans who disguised themselves as Dutchmen came to Japan as doctors employed by the Dutch East India Company. Caspar S. Schamberger from Leipzig stayed in Nagasaki in 1649, while Engelbert Kampher from Lomgo stayed there in 1690 [2]. As a surgeon, Schamberger founded the Casper-Ryu-Geka-Surgical Academy of Dutch Medicine in Nagasaki to train Japanese doctors. Kampher also practiced medicine, but he was better known as the first European author th publish a history of Japan in English. The book, entitled *The History of Japan*, was printed in London in 1727. While he was in Japan, Kampher, as a doctor accompanying a Dutch mission to the Shogun's government in Edo (now Tokyo), was granted an audience with the Shogun, Tsunayoshi Tokugawa.

Though Siebold's contribution to Japanese medicine was immeasurable, his academic achievement in introducing Japanese culture to Europe was equally significant. Siebold went far beyond Kampher's work in the field of Japanese studies, due in part to his self determination and personal effort favorable but also due to the attitude of the age, which was more than in the days when Kampher was in Japan some 130 years earlier.

Scholarly books were translated into Dutch from other European languages and they too came to Japan via Holland, along with the doctors. An anatomy book published in Dutch in 1723 was translated into Japanese by Genpaku Sugita and his colleagues in 1774. The book, entitled *Kaitai Shinsho* (New Book of Anatomy), was the most famous medical book ever introduced from Holland. The original book was the German *Anatomische Tabellen* written by a German named Johann Adam Kulmus.

Western medicine was taught in Nagasaki as part of "rangaku" (Dutch learning) or the study of western sciences in the Dutch language.. Particularly because surgery was a new field of medical treatment in Japan, the doctors at the Dutch factory were constantly asked by their Japanese counterparts to provide training.

Dejima in Nagasaki

In the seventeeth Century, Japan's feudal government in Edo closed the country, and prohibited Christianity in Japan. The government feared that Japan would be conquered by such Catholic countries as Portugal and Spain. By the early seventeenth century all trading relations with these Catholic countries were prohibited. However, because Holland was not considered to be a Catholic state, Dutch traders were allowed to come to Nagasaki and reside on a small island of Dejima (Fig. 2). The fan-shaped island was constructed in Nagasaki Harbor (Fig. 3) by the Tokugawa Shogunate in 1636. This 3.24-acre artificial land was the only place in Japan where Westerners, first the Portuguese and later the Dutch, were allowed to reside for the 218 years from 1636 to 1859, when Japan was reopened to the western world. In other words, Dejima was the only window through which western culture was introduced to Japan during the national seclusion period.

No Japanese other than government officials, a limited number of merchants, and courtesans were given access to De-

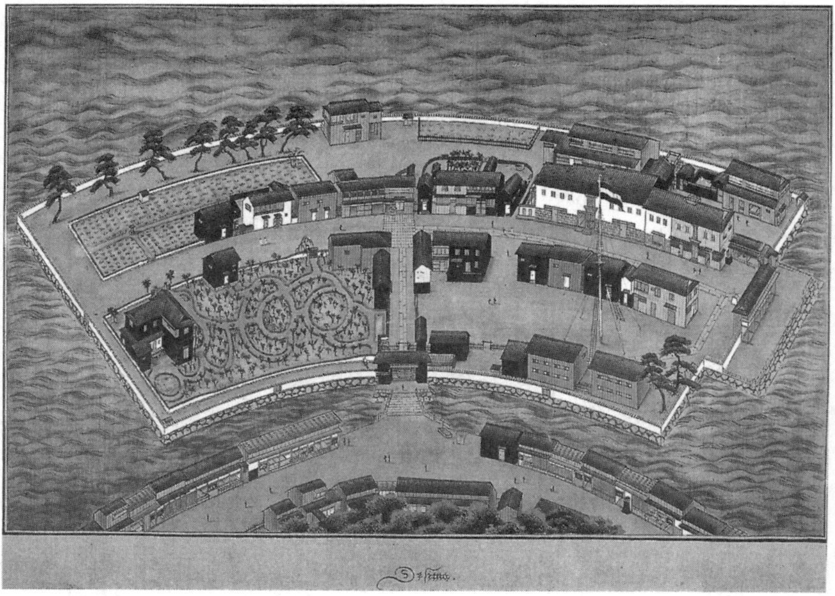

Fig. 2. The island of Dejima in the port of Nagasaki

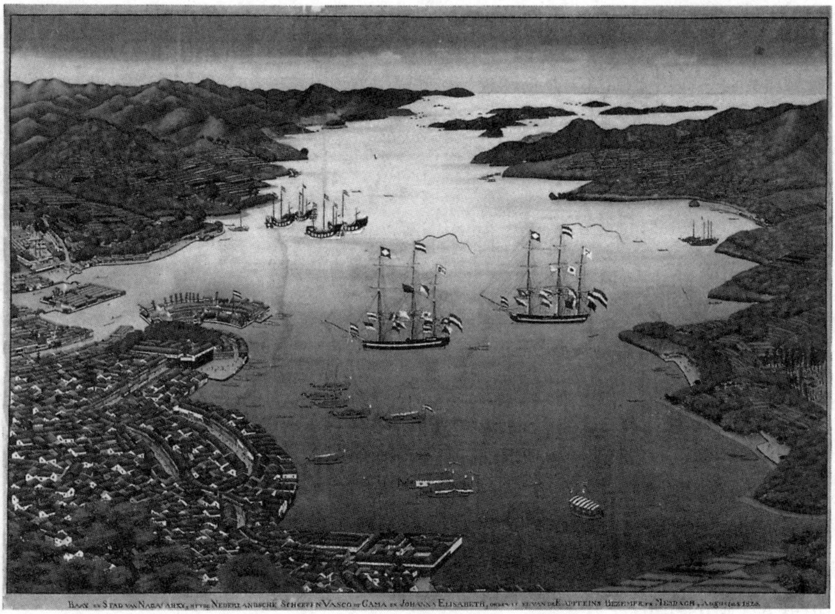

Fig. 3. The bay and city of Nagasaki, with ships of the Dutch East India Company

jima, while the Dutch were strictly prohibited from leaving Dejima without permission. One bridge was used to walk across to the island from the mainland. Warehouses, trading houses and living quarters were built on the island. Although the buildings were made of wood, they were all in western style and some botanical gardens were even added for the comfort of the Westerners.

Medical Treatment by Siebold

Siebold introduced European medical instruments, including those for orthopedics, obstetrics, dentistry and ophthalmology, and small portable instruments for surgery. Many are now preserved and displayed in the Nagasaki Prefectural Art Museum (Fig. 4). Treatment for cataracts was the first surgical procedure performed by Siebold. He also ordered a vaccine lymph of cowpox through the East India Company in order to perform vaccination, though it was spoiled and unusable on its arrival in Japan because it had been stored at a high temperature during ship-

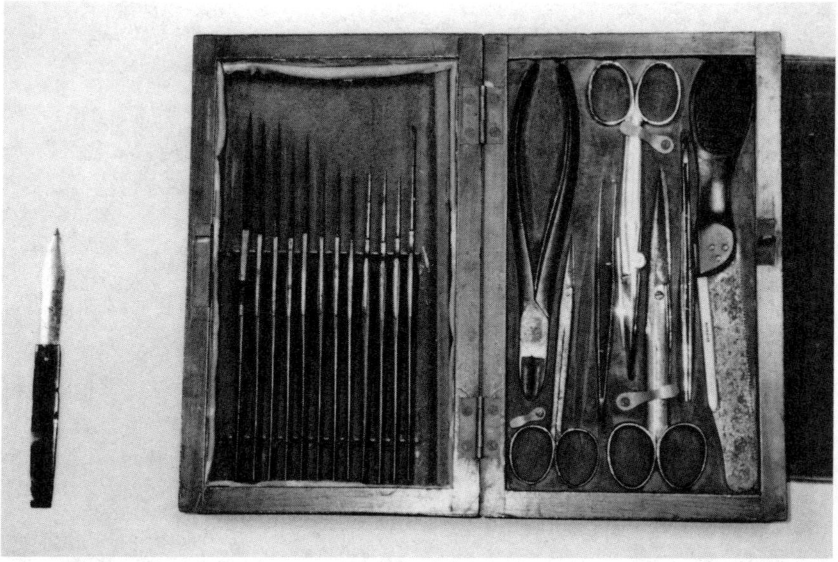

Fig. 4. Some of Siebold's medical instruments. (Courtesy of Nagasaki Prefectural Art Museum)

ment. However, it was helpful for teaching the general idea of vaccination to Japanese students.

Siebold's skillful surgical procedure won a reputation within the city of Nagasaki through government officials and merchants coming and going to Dejima. Soon, he was asked to perform medical treatment outside Dejima.

The name Siebold was pronounced "zi:bolt" in German, but he has been called "si:bolt" (as in the Dutch pronunciation) in Japan up to the present, which shows that he professed to be a Dutchman, not a German.

The name of this outstanding surgeon on Dejima became the talk of the town, especially among young Japanese doctors who gathered in Nagasaki to learn western medicine. Josef Kreiner, a professor of Japanese studies at Bonn University, once said that Siebold, as a young man of 27 and a recent graduate of a medical college, was very positive about his profession and this, with his intellectual curiosity and adventurous spirit, led to his success in Nagasaki.

Siebold possessed a curious mind, and was interested in all fields of natural science. In particular, he wanted to learn about

Japanese culture, the humanities, and the flora and fauna of Japan. However, he could not collect as many botanical and zoological samples as he wished on Dejima alone. Therefore, whenever possible, he tried to obtain these materials and information from visiting Japanese doctors in exchange for medical information from the western world.

In 1824, thanks to his fame and outstanding achievement as a doctor, Siebold was allowed to open a private school in the village of Narutaki in Nagasaki and to establish courses in clinical medicine while providing medical treatment. His Narutaki school is now the site of Nagasaki Municipal Siebold Memorial Hall (Fig. 5).

Siebold gave clinical lectures and established a herb garden at his school. With such famous Japanese doctors as Junzou Mima and Kenkai Oka in position as head teachers, he demonstrated practical methods and techniques in surgery, obstetrics and ophthalmology. Consequently, many doctors and patients came from all over the country [3].

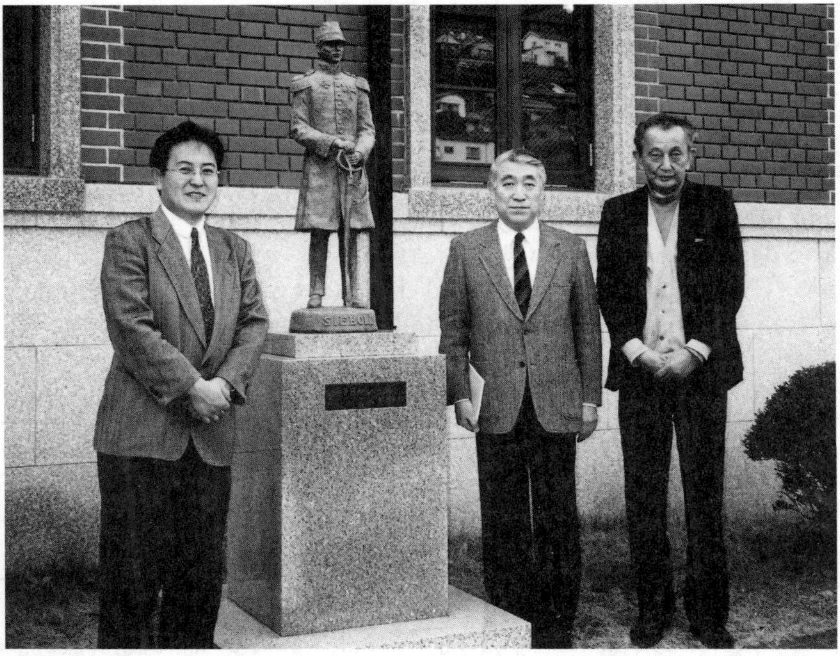

Fig. 5. Siebold's statue outside the Siebold Memorial Museum, with (*left* to *right*) Masahide Miyasaka, Yoshiki Hiki and Nakanishi

According to Professor Ogawa [3], Siebold used a very effective technique of training his students. He assigned various themes to them and told them to write their papers in Dutch. It is interesting to know that the German translation of Junzou Mima's paper was published in a journal of obstetrics in Frankfurt am Main, Germany, in 1826 under the title "Nippon Sanka Mondo" or "Questions and Answers in Japanese Obstetrics." Incidentally, Professor Ogawa wrote that Mima's article was the first Japanese paper ever to appear in a European professional journal.

Siebold conferred a doctor's license inscribed in his own writing in Dutch upon his graduating students (some of the documents are now stored in the Siebold Memorial Hall). Medical prescriptions in his own dutch writing are still to be found in Nagasaki. They date from the period 1823 to 1827, and were written with brushes on Japanese rice paper by Siebold himself. They were recorded in a notebook called "Siebold Kenpou-roku" which was kept by his students[1]. These records provide valuable insight into what kind of internal medicine was practiced by Siebold in those days.

Siebold's treatments are described in detail, with some brush-drawn illustrations, in the record entitled "A copy of direct transmission of remedies by Siebold and a corresponding diary of treatment"[2]. According to the records, Siebold commuted from Dejima to give these treatments.

Records of the treatment given by Siebold and his students for oscheoedema, harelip, cerebral edema, leg injuries, fractures and orthopedic surgery for facial wounds caused by syphilis were also described in the Diary[4, 5].

Procedures for the surgical treatment of a case of cerebral edema were also described in detail, with illustrations (Fig. 6).

---

[1] Students of Siebold: Siebold Kenpo-roku, the record of medical examination and treatment. The date of the original document is unknown and it is currently missing, although a copy is stored in the Siebold Memorial Hall.

[2] Students of Siebold: The copy of direct transmission of remedies by Siebold and the corresponding diary of treatment: Tenri library complete books, vol. 80, collection of manuscripts of scholars of western learning, Yagi-shoten, 1986, Tokyo.

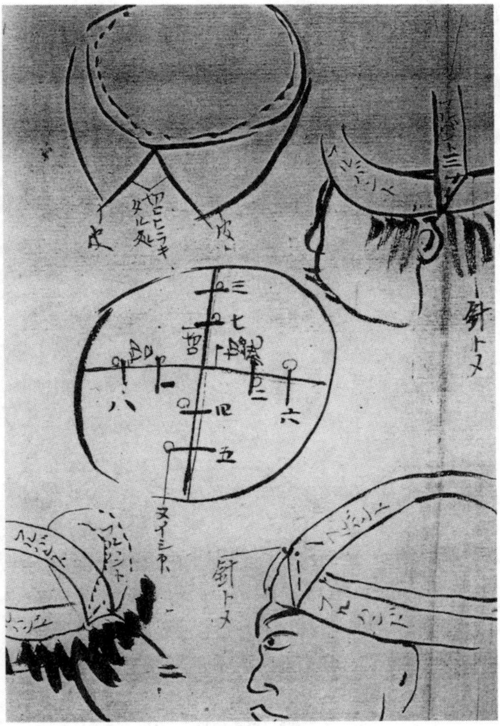

Fig. 6. Illustrations for an operation by Siebold on a cranial tumor

Removing a cranial tumor was quite a serious procedure at that time. The patient was a 12-year- old boy from a Samurai family. It was recorded, however, that the boy underwent surgery without anesthesia and endured the painful operation without crying or screaming. The surgery was performed by Siebold and his assistant doctor from the Dutch factory, and Japanese students took care of the patient after the initial operation. The patient urinated right after the operation. The boy was hungry and was orally given some laudanum and digitalis dissolved in rice soup. Two days later, the boy had a bowel movement and the operation was thought to be successful. However, the patient died of fever 4 days later.

Illustrations of facial sutures used in orthopedic surgery showed that Paré's suture was used for facial wounds caused by the syphilis which raged throughout the country in those days. It is of interest that these suture illustrations were similar to those

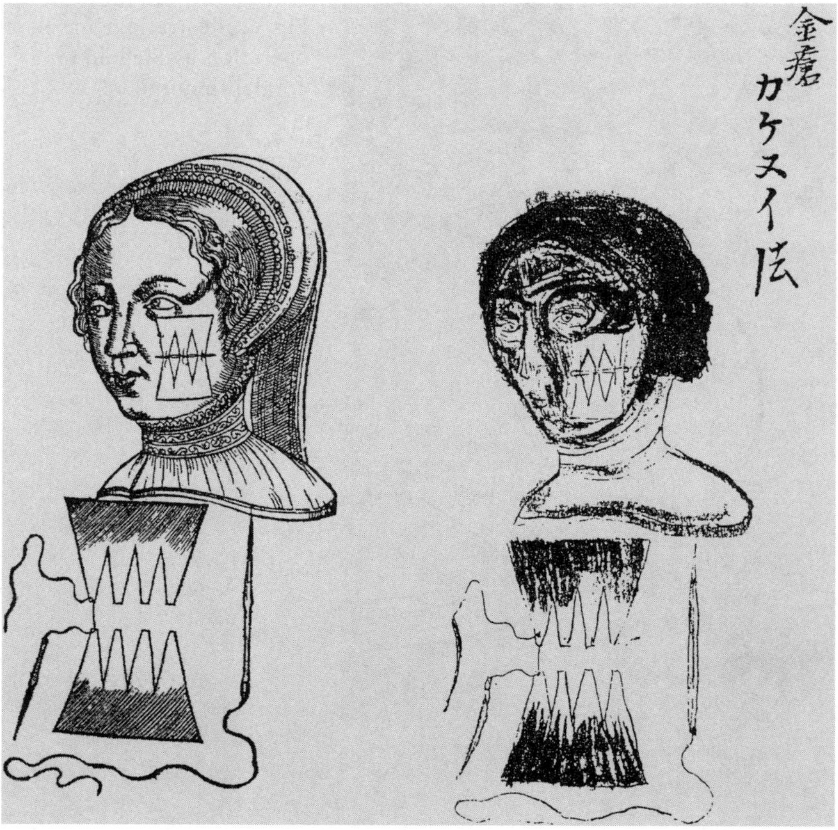

Fig. 7. Facial suture methods by Ambroise Paré (*left*) and Philipp Franz von Siebold (*right*)

appearing in a surgical book by Paré which had already been introduced to Japan. We wonder if Siebold ever actually performed Paré's suture (Fig. 7).

Siebold was expelled from Japan at the end of December 1829, as he was allegedly suspected of being involved in spying against Japan and of trying to smuggle out of the country documents that were forbidden to be removed under the seclusion policy. Thus he returned to Europe. However, he could not forget his affection for Japan. He subsequently returned to Japan and stayed for about 3 years from 1859 to 1862. During his second stay he somehow practiced medicine again, as shown by the later

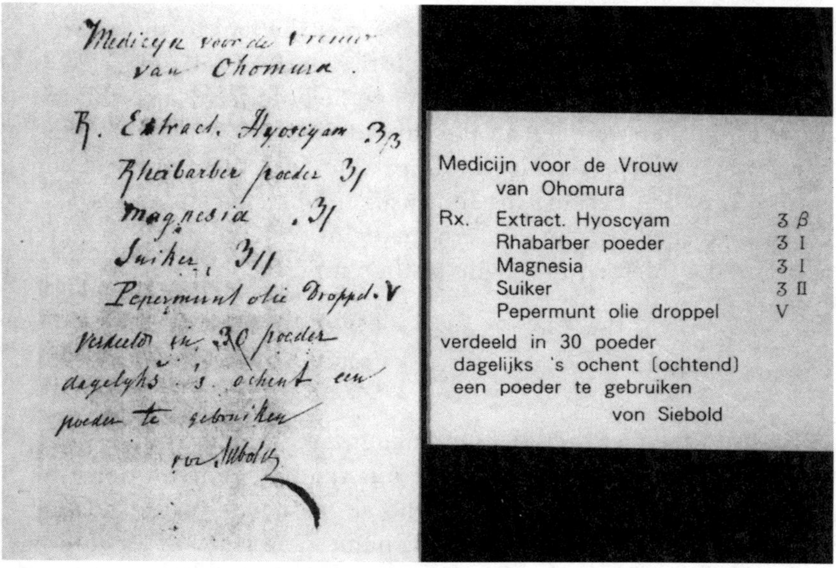
Medicijn voor de Vrouw
van Ohomura
Rx. Extract. Hyoscyam ʒ β
Rhabarber poeder ʒ I
Magnesia ʒ I
Suiker ʒ II
Pepermunt olie droppel V
verdeeld in 30 poeder
dagelijks 's ochent (ochtend)
een poeder te gebruiken
von Siebold

Fig. 8. One of Siebold's prescriptions

discovery of some prescriptions in his own writing, of which Itsuo Miyazaki made a detailed study[4, 5] (Fig. 8).

Though Siebold continued to practice medicine, he did not conduct any furthur medical training for Japanese doctors, which was rather a surprise for the people who knew him earlier. We-can only infer that either Siebold's interest in medicine had declined or that he thought his professional ability and skill as a doctor had declined. At the same time, he was devoting much of his time to studying things Japanese, and was probably not keeping abreast of progress in European medicine. He may have thought that he could no longer offer anything new to his Japanese counterparts.

Siebold left a vital legacy. He trained numerous Japanese doctors at his medical school, and many of them are well remembered in Japanese medical history as they continued their activities as doctors, scholars, and medical researchers throughout Japan.

At this point, we must mention Siebold's child. It was said that a woman named Taki was one of the patients treated by Siebold and that she later became his wife. Young Siebold fell in love with 16-year-old Taki when he saw her. However, since only courtesans were allowed to enter Dejima, she had to stay there with Siebold as a courtesan, though they were legally married. They had a daughter called Ine. When Siebold left Nagasaki, Ine and her mother were left in the care of Siebold's students. One such student was Keisaku Ninomiya who gave Ine a medical education; Ine then became the first woman obstetrician and gynecologist to specialize in western medicine in Japan. She was later appointed a doctor to the wife of the Emperor Meiji [6].

Conclusion

Despite the fact that Siebold encountered many troubles and difficulties in Japan, he made outstanding contributions to Japan as a doctor. We Japanese who are associated with the medical profession will never forget his name. The story of Siebold is still told from generation to generation, even among Japanese laymen. Siebold is without a doubt the most famous foreign doctor in the history of Japan.

Acknowledgements

We acknowledge the valuable support and advice of Professor Toshiro Omura of Keio University, the authority on the history of the medical sciences, who kindly read this article and offered many helpful suggestions.

References

1. Morioka Y, Omura T (1991) Paré, father of modern surgery. NHK books, Tokyo
2. Kraas E, Hiki Y (eds) (1992) 300 years of Japanese-German interchanges in medicine [300 Jahre deutsch-japanische Beziehungen in der Medizin]. Springer, Berlin Heidelberg New York
3. Ogawa T (1964) The history of medicine. Chuo-Koron, Tokyo
4. Miyazaki I (1991) Das Rezept (die Rezepte) von Siebold [in Japanese]. J Hist Sci Jpn Pharmacol 26(1):12–23
5. Miyazaki I (1995) Das Rezept (die Rezepte) von Siebold [in Japanese]. J Hist Sci Jpn Pharmacol 30(2):116–124
6. Hiki S (1992) Mutige Frauen in einer Zeit ohne Frauenrecht. In: Kraas E, Hiki Y (eds) 300 Jahre deutsch-japanische Beziehungen in der Medizin. Springer, Berlin Heidelberg New York, pp 32–35

CHAPTER 7

On the Trail of the Siebold Family in Würzburg

U. Beireis, W. Klein-Langner

Traces of the Siebold family in Würzburg – many a Würzburg citizen will be able to lead a guest in this town to the Siebold-straße, Sieboldshöhe, a Siebold monument, the Siebold-Gymnasium (secondary school), and perhaps even to the more recent Siebold Museum. Those traces are easy for a stranger to find on the city map. The places where the Siebold family lived and operated in Würzburg are rather more hidden, however, and fewer people know about them. We wish to invite you, therefore, to join a Würzburg tour "on the trail of the Siebold family".

Our tour starts with baroque Würzburg and with the nineteenth century, which was the time when the Siebolds worked at the Juliusspital. This hospital occupies almost all of the upper left side of the Juliuspromenade, between the medieval part of Würzburg and the famous vineyards of Stein. It was founded by the counter-reformatory Prince Bishop Julius Echter von Mespelbrunn (1573–1617). After 4 years of construction, it was inaugurated on 10 July 1580 as a donation for "any sort of poor, ill, infirm, even injured people, needing medical care, and abandoned orphans, and pilgrims passing by, and needy persons"[1].

Soon, despite several disastrous fires, it became an important city hospital. Consequently, with the foundation of the medical faculty in 1593, medical university education was provided at the Juliusspital. This close relationship lasted until the university hospital of Luitpold-Krankenhaus was built (1912–1922).

Here at the Juliusspital, the Siebold family started their activities in Würzburg. In 1760, the "subsurgeon" Carl Caspar Siebold arrived in the city and studied medicine here; after a study

[1] Thomas Heiler, Das Weingut und Krankenhaus Juliusspital, in: Bayerisches Kulturmosaik, 1/97, p. 60.

trip to Paris, Rouen, London, and Leiden, as a result of his professional skills, he advanced to the position of assistant surgeon and later senior surgeon at the Juliusspital. From 1769, Carl Caspar was also professor of medicine and lectured on anatomy, surgery, and obstetrics.

His contemporary Carl Gottfried Scharold says of Carl Caspar's work that he "attracted many students of surgery by his important and successful operations in Franconia and all over Germany; his school is unsurpassed in this country, and the Charité in Berlin as well as the famous Josephsspital in Vienna can equal it, at best. Many really clever and great surgeons have been formed there"[2].

At the same Juliusspital, Carl Caspar and his sons Christoph, Barthel, and Elias (the latter two had been called back from their studies in Jena) treated the injured from the battle near Würzburg in 1796. They saved hundreds of lives by this action, including 577 Austrians and at least 200 French. Their efforts earned them hereditary nobility in 1801.

Through the gateway we enter the inner court of the building. Do not miss taking a look at the ancient pharmacy of the Juliusspital. We cross the court and go to the right. There is a door plate at the entrance. Under Prince Bishop Adam Friedrich von Seinsheim, this pharmacy was established between 1760 and 1765. The original equipment is preserved, including shelves, wood carvings, frescos, and stucco works. This is the ambiance where the Siebolds worked.

When Carl Caspar was lecturing it became clear that, for regular instruction, a theatrum anatomicum was needed. Siebold obviously pestered his principal so regularly that he agreed to reorganize the building, and the anatomy theater was inaugurated on 9 July 1788. We reach this building on passing through the Fürstenbau (prince's edifice). It is the baroque pavilion on the right in the garden planned by Joseph Greising and built between 1705 and 1714. The medical faculty of the University of Würzburg had been using this building since 1726. The two statues at the northern front are by Johann Peter Wagner. One represents an anatomist with a skull, the other a physician pointing at a heart and a

[2] Carl Gottfried Scharold, Würzburg und die umliegende Gegend, Stahel, Würzburg, 1805, p. 255.

lobe of the lung. Carl Caspar was wise enough to put the reconstruction of this pavilion in its true light by publishing a manuscript "On the Advantages of a Public Anatomic School for the State", in which he fully explained the construction and layout of "his" anatomy: "Anatomic schools are the most beneficial institutions a sovereign can establish for his subjects"[3].

A short time later, however, the pavilion was reconstructed again. The new professor of anatomy, Johann Friedrich Fuchs, who came from the university of Jena, found fault with the lighting and the limited capacity of the auditorium[4]. Nowadays this garden pavilion is mainly used for cultural events.

Now we leave the Juliusspital and turn towards another very modern institution originated by the Siebold family. We walk back to the Juliuspromenade and turn right towards the Main river. At the monument for the founder of the Juliusspital, we turn left into Dominikanerplatz. A few steps further at the right a lane called Innerer Graben begins. This name indicates the former inner moat of the medieval fortifications.

Following the lane, we reach a rather inconspicuous, green-plastered house with the number 16. This is the former Freihaus (free house) with the old name of IInd district, no. 135/136. Its small bay-window has an epigraph commemorating Christoph Siebold, who founded a maternity home here to remedy the grievance that single pregnant women were left without medical assistance. This extremely modern institution[5] was inaugurated on 17 December 1791. Carl Gottfried Scharold reports again:

---

[3] Carl Caspar von Siebold, Rede von den Vortheilen, welche der Staat durch öffentliche anatomische Lehranstalten gewinnt, Nürnberg 1788, p. 7.

[4] See Robert Herrlinger, Wiedergefundene Pläne der Anatomie im Juliusspital aus dem Jahre 1804, in: Die Mainlande 9, 1958, 14:53–56.

[5] The *Frankfurter Allgemeine Zeitung* printed a reported on 15 April 1997 (p. 13) about "Europe's first obstetric house in Berlin" and its tenth anniversary: "Many ideas, such as rooming in and the parturition stool, have been adopted by hospitals. The midwives are proud to report on very well attended training courses for hospital midwives about 'positions during parturition'". Obviously, the knowledge imparted by the Siebold family in Würzburg 200 years ago, and later in Berlin by Elias von Siebold, has to be reacquired laboriously in modern times.

> This school is most important for mankind and owes its origin to the electoral senior officer of health Carl Caspar von Siebold, the Nestor of this university. His son, the early deceased Professor Christoph von Siebold, raised it to an academic school and made every effort to preserve a maternity home as well as to improve constantly his lectures.

A temporary maternity hospital was installed in the free house in the Innerer Graben which was owned by the municipal authorities and usually assigned to the senior city midwife. The police used this house to accommodate accident victims, though these were mainly pregnant country wives who were surprised by their labor-pains when selling their vegetables at the market and could not reach their home village. The midwife who lived here also took in pregnant women. Notwithstanding its limitations, it produced within a short period of time many obstetricians who are appreciated and famous in Germany. The house was sufficient to accommodate seven pregnant women and had an average of 24–30 deliveries per year. With the professor's improved equipment, the house usually accommodated nine or ten pregnant women; however, as well as other drawbacks, it was too small for its intended use by the police as well as acting as an academic school. The allowance offered to pregnant women consisted of accommodation, bed, firewood and medicine. All other requirements, e.g., the charges for baptism and legal registration, were covered by the contributions of the regular students[6].

Now we continue our tour in the same direction toward the riverside and at the crossroads turn right, back to the Juliuspromenade. At the end of the promenade on the left we see the Alter Kranen (old crane) in front of us. Before reaching it we turn left into Karmelitenstraße, where number 20 is called Rückermainhof. This town palace was built by Joseph Greising in 1715–1722. It is a place of major importance in the scientific education of the later explorer of Japan Philipp Franz von Siebold. He wrote in a letter to his uncle Elias in Berlin, dated 16 July 1818:

---

[6] Carl Gottfried Scharold, Würzburg 1805, p. 221 f.

"For one and a half years now I have been lodging with the prosector and privy councillor Doellinger, who will certainly guide my education to your satisfaction. Almost every day he is surveying my work in anatomy, botanics and therapeutics ..."[7]. The professor's flat was on the first floor. The all-round education Siebold received here in his professor's flat in Würzburg undoubtedly prepared him for his later research activity in Japan in almost every branch of the natural sciences.

Now we go back a few steps and turn right into the Marktgasse (market lane). The parish register mentions that Philipp Franz's parents, Professor Christoph Siebold and his wife Apollonia, lived here. Probably the birthplace of the explorer of Japan was in this street, known then as Maingasse. Unfortunately, the register does not mention the house number.

Let us turn to the right and midway up the lane go past the romanesque doorway of the famous and oldest wine restaurant of Würzburg, Zum Stachel, towards the market place. Straight ahead, where now we see the grey ventilation system of the garage under the market square, the house Zum Vögelein, IInd district, no. 433, once stood. Later, the address was renamed as Marktplatz 4. This was the former dwelling house of Elias von Siebold, youngest son of Carl Caspar von Siebold and professor of obstetrics in Würzburg and Berlin. Its ruins from the last war have been completely pulled down.

We now cross the marketplace, go past the Marienkapelle (St. Mary's Chapel) and the Falkenhaus (house of the hawk) and turn right into the Kürschnerhof (furriers' yard). After passing the front of the Neumünster church, a few steps further, we arrive in front of the historic and spiritual center of Würzburg, the Kiliansdom (St. Kilian's Cathedral).

The bishopric of Würzburg was founded by Bonifatius in 742. It became one of the most important political centers of the German Reich during the Middle Ages. The cathedral is connected to the Siebold family through the usual church ceremonies, such as the wedding of Carl Caspar and Margarethe Veron-

[7] Auf den Spuren Siebolds in Würzburg und Japan, catalogue of the inaugural exhibition of the Siebold Museum, Udo Beireis and Jorinde Ebert (eds) Siebold-Gesellschaft, Würzburg, 1995, p. 21.

ica Stang on 15 July 1766 (she was the daughter of her husband's predecessor and professor at the Juliusspital, the surgeon Christoph Stang). In the same cathedral their first son Christoph and their grandson Philipp Franz were baptized. We should therefore have a look at the preserved baptismal font. We enter the cathedral through the main door and turn to the right. Two romanesque columns flank the entrance of the baptistery. This baptismal font is the only major cast-iron work from the thirteenth century in Southern Germany. It was created by Master Eckard from Worms in 1279 and its eight reliefs represent the history of salvation.

We leave the cathedral by the main door again and turn to the left in Plattnerstraße, which then bends to the left and leads to Domerschulstraße. We continue to the right and reach the so-called Alte Universität (Old University) on the left. This building complex has been called "old" since the "New University" was built at Sanderring in 1897. The present university was founded by Prince Bishop Julius Echter on 2 January 1582.

We turn left along Domerschulstraße and reach the main gateway of the Old University. There we can admire a relief with the inscription *Die Sendung des heiligen Geistes* (Holy Ghost Mission), who, according to the founder's wish, was to regulate university life. This is the place where, besides Carl Caspar, the Siebolds who followed him had their academic training: Barthel from 1793 to 1797 (continued at Jena), Elias from 1792 to 1795 (Jena 1795–1797, Göttingen 1797–1798) and Philipp Franz from 1815 to 1820. Christoph had been to Altdorf and Göttingen universities, and after 1 year in Würzburg Damian changed to Göttingen in 1789.

Philipp Franz began his studies of philosophy in the winter semester 1815/16. Unfortunately, his thesis has been lost, but the family still holds the minutes of examination by Professor Ruland with the entry: "5th sept. 1820 the student Philipp Franz von Siebold from Würzburg, in his oral examination, was given the mark EXCELLENT by the majority"[8].

With Siebold's later success in his academic training in mind, we can now walk to its origins. We go back to the corner

[8] Auf den Spuren Siebolds, Würzburg 1995, p. 22.

of Domerschulstraße and then go left into Schönthalstraße. At the traffic lights, to the left we can see the impressive red sandstone building of Neubaukirche, now the university auditorium, used in Siebold's time for graduation examinations. Further on to the right Peterstraße begins, with the Peterplatz and the church of Saints Peter and Paul with its striking baroque front and romanesque body. Close to it is Münzstraße no. 1, today the seat of adult education. Here there used to be one of Würzburg's four Latin schools, the first essential of secondary schools and universities. The secondary school and university did not separate until 1794. Philipp Franz attended the Königliches Gymnasium zu Würzburg (royal secondary school), today called the Wirsberg-Gymnasium[9]. As we know that Philipp Franz lived with his uncle Lotz at Heidingsfeld from 1808, he probably went to the Latin school in Münzstraße, as this was the closest for him to reach on his way from Heidingsfeld. (Anyone interested in the history of this house may study the frescos in the passage under the splendid baroque gateway.)

Now we go back to the lane between the church and Münzstraße 1 and immediately come to the modern building of the regional government of Unterfranken (Lower Franconia). Passing the main doorway, we cross a small park. In front of us we see the Hexenturm (witch tower), the present university cashier's office. To the right, between the New University and the law court, there is a green island where we find the monument to Philipp Franz von Siebold. During the World Exposition in Vienna in 1873, the international gardeners' congress decided to honor the expert on Japan with a monument. Donations were collected from Austria, the Netherlands, Japan, and Germany. Professor Christoph Roth from Munich was charged with creating the bronze bust, which was unveiled on 8 October 1882 in the presence of Philipp Franz's sons Alexander and Heinrich, who were active diplomats in Japan.

If we continue our way in the same direction as before, after crossing the park of the former fortification and turning right into the next street, we reach the beginning of Sieboldstraße.

---

[9] The Corps Moenania preserves two copies of the annual report 1813/14 and 1814.

This street leads high up the hill named Sieboldshöhe. At the end are the Siebold-Anlagen (gardens), also called Siebold-Wäldchen (grove). There, in Hans-Löffler-Straße, Friedrich Karl von Siebold, the last of this name formally inaugurated a fountain in memory of his great ancestor in 1982.

Nowadays, however, the upper part of Sieboldstraße has been renamed Zeppelinstraße. This union of names in one street also describes a family history. The son of a Siebold daughter (Helene), Alexander von Brandenstein, married the only daughter of the airship builder, Graf Ferdinand von Zeppelin, in 1909[10].

The von Brandenstein-Zeppelin family feels close to both branches of this family.

Now, however, let us continue on Ottostraße past the lawcourt, toward the town center. On the right side of the street we see the long building of Kilianeum, Ottostraße 3. This is the former St. Afra cloister, secularized in 1803. This is where Elias von Siebold originally tried to install an obstetric hospital. Soon, however, he was offered a better building and the plan was abandoned.

Via Ottostraße and Balthasar Neumann Promenade we reach the Residenz, the ancient summer residence of the Prince Bishops of Würzburg. This edifice was inaugurated in 1743 when the Hofkirche (the court church) was consecrated by Prince Bishop Friedrich Carl von Schönborn.

The connecting street between the Residenz and the cathedral is Hofstraße. Following this street a few steps, we reach the courtyard of the Mozart-Gymnasium, which has some further Siebold traces. In 1858 this was an agricultural and commercial school, later named Maxschule. In this school Philipp Franz von Siebold installed his first Japanisches Museum for public exhibition from 1865 until 1866 (Würzburg's first Siebold museum)[11].

---

[10] For further information see Udo Beireis, The Brandenstein-Zeppelin family – 100 years family possessions in the castle of Brandenstein, in: Ausstellungskatalog zum 200. Geburtstag Philipp Franz von Siebolds, Nagasaki 1996, pp. 24–29.

[11] The Würzburg Siebold Museum was inaugurated in 1995 and it welcomes you at Frankfurter Straße 87, in the former villa of the directors of a brewery.

There he exhibited a collection from his second journey to Japan, 1859–1863. This collection was sold to the State of Bavaria in 1874 and is now integrated into the Völkerkundemuseum (ethnologic museum) of Munich[12]. Even later on, this school did not give up its ties to von Siebold. In this building the Realgymnasium (secondary school) was inaugurated on 8 October 1864. In 1907, this school moved to Rennweger Ring 11, and in 1961 it was renamed the Siebold-Gymnasium[13].

From Hofstraße we turn right into Maxstraße, the former main entrance to the Maxschule. Then we follow this street as far as Kardinal-Faulhaber-Platz, opposite the municipal theater. At the traffic lights we turn left into Theaterstraße. During the 1740s, due to the expansion of the fortification walls, the medieval town-moat was filled up and new houses were built on these sites. The street was called "Auf dem Graben" (on the moat) and was renamed Theaterstraße in 1840[14]. In the house at Theaterstraße 8 (Äußerer Graben 75, II District)[15] Carl Caspar had his apartment.

Further in this direction, Theaterstraße runs into Barbarossaplatz with a left branch to Oberthürstraße. This was the home of Barthel von Siebold. The former name of the building was Obere Wöllergasse 6, II District, No. 81[16].

When we turn to the right in the Barbarossaplatz, we see the magnificent facade of Stift Haug. This church is the main masterpiece of the baroque architect Antonio Petrini (1625–1701), was destroyed in 1945 and its interior is now rather plain. It was the church where the brothers Damian, Barthel, and Elias were baptized. Barthel married here on 25 August 1799 and Christoph

[12] See Udo Beireis, Die zweite japanische Sammlung des Philipp Franz von Siebold, in: Mainländer Nachrichten, special edition August 1996, ed. Corps Moenania, Würzburg.

[13] Werner Dettelbacher, Jahresbericht des Siebold-Gymnasiums 1966/67 (annual grammar school report).

[14] Hans Körner, Die Würzburger Siebold, Eine Gelehrtenfamilie des 18. und 19. Jahrhunderts, Neustadt an der Aisch, 1966, p. 495.

[15] Vollständiges Adreß-Buch, der Chur. Haupt- und Residenzstadt Würzburg, Stahel, Würzburg, 1806, p. 208.

[16] Vollständiges Adreß-Buch, Würzburg, 1806, p. 208.

Siebold was buried in its churchyard on 18 January 1798. This churchyard, however, no longer exists[17].

Close to this church, towards the railway station, is the Matthias-Ehrenfried-Haus, with the Matrikelamt of Würzburg (register office). This place preserves the first official sign of life of the explorer of Japan: the parish register of the cathedral with the entry on Philipp Franz[18].

Following Bahnhofstraße in the same direction, we finally reach on the left a house with the former name of Teufelstorgasse I District, No. 230, today Bahnhofstraße 9. Here was where the much-traveled, world-famous explorer moved into an apartment in Würzburg for the last time. After long years outside Würzburg, at Leiden, Leiderdorp, St. Boppard, and Bonn, Philipp Franz von Siebold moved into this house in spring 1864, welcomed by a torchlight procession of "his" Corps Moenania (a duelling student's fraternity). Siebold had joined this students' fraternity as member number 18 in 1816 and was much attached to it all his life. The first portrait of Siebold is an album leaf showing him smoking and drinking beer during a joyful party[19]. The fraternity's tradition reports that Siebold fought 33 duels during his studies. The scars he received acquired for him, during his first stay in Japan as a young physician, the fame of a samurai.

[17] After her husband died in 1798, the widow Apollonia von Siebold, née Lotz, moved to her brother's home in Heidingsfeld, beyond Würzburg's town gates, in 1809. This brother was a parson and, from 1821, a member of the Würzburg cathedral chapter. She kept house for him for "more than 30 years" (according to the last will of Franz Josef Lotz, ed. E. von Soder-Güldenstubbe, WDGBL 57, 1995, p. 375). When he died, Apollonia lived in Martinsgasse 5, between 1838 and 1841 at Vor dem Sandertore (Körner, p. 558, Anm. 42). In 1845, Philipp Franz called his mother to Leiderdorp, where she died soon afterwards.

[18] Diocese archives, Matrikelamt, Matthias-Ehrenfried-Haus, 1, VIII, 1782–1811, p. 337.

[19] Philipp Franz von Siebold's memory is cherished up to the present day by this students' fraternity. On the occasion of his 200th anniversary, a reception was given on the premises of this fraternity (Mergentheimer Straße 14) in the presence of Mayor Ito of Nagasaki and Mayor Weber of Würzburg.

In April 1866, Siebold moved to Munich in order to exhibit his Japanese collection and persuade the State of Bavaria to acquire it. This is where Siebold died on 18 October 1866[20].

Now we walk to the end of the street and turn left, along the Kaiserplatz, across Kaiserstraße, into Marcusstraße and Klinikstraße. At Klinikstraße 6 there was formerly a house that was used for epileptic patients from 1775 until 1805. In 1805 Elias von Siebold, who was also a gynecologist, succeeded in installing a maternity hospital here. Later it became an ophthalmology sanatorium and from 1901 to 1922 it belonged to the gynecological hospital[21].

A contemporary describes the maternity hospital as follows:

It is a three stories high building. In the ground floor, in addition to the economic facilities, there are a dining room and a workroom for the pregnant women at free board as well as three dormitories with three beds each one. In the second floor, there is a spacious auditorium, a delivery room with an amphitheater for students and midwives, one adjacent waiting room for students, two major maternity rooms with three beds and three minor maternity rooms with two beds as well as two tiny with one bed each for venereal diseases and infections. In the third floor there are several rooms for household facilities, three major and well furnished rooms for paying patients of the upper classes and one room in which Elias v. Siebold's own collection of obstetric instruments, bowls, specimens, drawings, copper plate prints and anatomical models are stored.

In this same street Professor Elias von Siebold had a second dwelling house at Klinikstraße 10 (Oberwallgasse 269), where he

[20] The tomb, in which his wife Helene von Gagern also found her last resting-place, is on view in the Alter Südlicher Friedhof (ancient southern cemetery) in Munich, section 33, row 13, no. 5.

[21] Thomas Memminger, Würzburger Straßen und Bauten, Würzburg, Geb. Memminger, 1921, p. 227.

[22] C.F.L. Wildberg, Jahrbuch der Universitäten Deutschlands, 1810, p. 334f.

lived until he moved to Berlin in April 1816. Today it houses the university institute of mathematics.

When we now follow this street in the same direction, we come back to the starting point of our tour, to the Juliusspital.

CHAPTER 8

Philipp Franz von Siebold and His Influence on the Cultural Development of Japan

M. Miyasaka

Philipp Franz Siebold, the Japan investigator from Würzburg, had his 200th anniversary last year. On this occasion Würzburg and several towns in Japan organized an extensive exhibition of his work. Furthermore, in Tokyo and Osaka a huge exhibition of Siebold's Nippon collection was supported by the German institute for investigations in Japan and attended by more than 170,000 visitors[1].

Obviously, Japan did much more than Germany to honor the memory of Philipp Franz von Siebold. Japan did not forget the advantages Siebold won for his adopted country. I would suggest that Siebold is one of the most famous Germans ever to have visited Japan.

His life has been much explored. In 1986 the bibliography at Bochum University comprised 882 western and 740 Japanese titles on Siebold[2]. Since then more titles have probably been added. However, his lifelong interest in Japan has not yet been completely explored: scattered all over Europe, many documents on or by him have not yet been analyzed. His descendants, the Brandenstein-Zeppelin family, alone have more than 7000 documents. The Siebold Memorial Museum in Nagasaki began an analysis in 1990[3].

---

[1] According to the statistics of the Edo Tokyo museum and the national museum for ethnology in Osaka.

[2] Eschbach-Szabo, Kneider H (eds) (1986) Acta Sieboldiana II, Siebold-Bibliographie, Schriften über Philipp Franz von Siebold 1824–1984. Wiesbaden.

[3] Concerning the extent of documents in the castle of Brandenstein, see Miyasaka M (1996) Entstehung und Aufbau des Siebold-Archivs auf Burg Brandenstein. In: Kreiner J (ed) Die Japansammlungen Philipp Franz und Heinrich von Siebolds, Miscellanea, No. 12, Deutsches Institut für Japanstudien, Tokyo, pp. 70–80.

In the near future, Siebold will appear to us in another light, once those documents have been explored. Our present view of Siebold is composed, however, of three fields of activities:

1. By teaching western medicine to Japanese physicians, Siebold initiated modern medical science in Japan.
2. Siebold was the first to apply modern scientific research methods in Japan and, by explaining his results, he depicted a correct view of Japan for Europe.
3. Siebold was politically engaged and thus won the sympathy of Europe for Japan (something which is less well known nowadays).

The merit I mentioned first was the transfer of western medical knowledge to Japan. He initiated modern medical development in Japan. Many Japanese know this and venerate him deeply. How was this possible for a young man of 27 who, after his medical studies in Würzburg, had practiced for a short time in Heidingsfeld but was not a very experienced physician?

It was from the Dutch factory on Dejima that the Japanese heard about Siebold's arrival in Japan in 1823. He had been announced as a great physician. More than 50 Japanese physicians met in Nagasaki in order to learn about recent western medicine from him. His modern education at Würzburg University meant that Siebold's knowledge of the practice and theory of diagnosis and treatment had been completed by a solid education in minor medical subjects such as botany and pharmacology.

In Siebold's time, more and more Japanese scientists wished to learn more than fragmentary information about western research. They asked for systematic and extended knowledge about "rangaku", the so-called Dutch science, and Siebold was qualified to impart it. Thus the first transfer of modern medical education to Japan originated in Würzburg, Bavaria.

After the breakdown of the Tokugawa shogunate in 1867, the new Meji government introduced German methods of medical education. It is small wonder, therefore, that Shutôjo, the first government institute for smallpox vaccination in Japan that preceded the Imperial University of Tokyo was founded with the cooperation of two disciples of Siebold.

Incidentally, Siebold was one of those who initiated smallpox vaccination in Japan. In a letter to his uncle Adam Elias von

Siebold in Berlin Siebold wrote, as a postscript: "I introduced the vaccines in Japan". This letter dates back to 1823[4].

Scientific research was not Siebold's main task at Dejima; instead it was the medical care of the factory workers. In addition, the factory physician undertook scientific research and studies of Japan. Siebold was not the only one to do this; his predecessors, such as the German Engelbert Kämpfer from Lemgo (1651–1716) and the Swede Karl Peter Thunberg from Uppsala (1743–1828), had done the same. All of them made detailed observations and reports on Japan. The "three scientists of Dejima", as they are called in Japan, were interested not only in medicine but also in other natural sciences.

Europe was particularly interested in the results found by those well informed men. Due to the Tokugawa shogunate's politics of isolation little information existed about Japan. Furthermore, the observation and exploration of an unexplored land, as Japan was, must have been an attractive quest for every scientist. However, Siebold was much more successful than his predecessors. In addition, he profited from the Dutch government's plan to improve the poor commercial relationship between the Netherlands and Japan. For this Holland needed good scientific knowledge about the economic possibilities of that unexplored country. For appropriate research work Siebold received considerable financial support. This was the basis for an extended exploration of Japan, as we can see from Siebold's collections and his work. His collection of Japanese everyday objects from the Edo period, particularly, is unrivaled in quality and quantity. In Japan, no such collection exists. People used to throw away old shoes, clothes, brooms and so on.

Siebold even had many Japanese disciples. He charged them with scientific problems and thus taught them European scientific methods. Through Siebold's instruction his disciples discovered not only the importance of western medicine but also that of modern science itself. He wrote to his uncle Adam Elias von Siebold in Berlin in 1827 "The light of science expands all over Japan from the small valley of Narutaki". And this was not at all exaggerated. Then, due to the so-called "Siebold affair",

[4] Körner H (1967) Die Würzburger Siebold, eine Gelehrtenfamilie des 18. und 19. Jahrhunderts. Neustadt a. d. Aisch, p. 822.

Philipp Franz von Siebold was banished from Japan. Consequently, western science was suppressed, and so were the Japanese scientists who had been working with it.

Chouei Takano from Mizusawa (1804–1850), one of Siebold's closest disciples, published a book on "Bojutsu Yumemonogatari" in which he warned about the dangerous western influence in eastern Asia, saying that Asia could not cope with highly advanced western technology. Chouei Takano suggested, therefore, that more intense study of western science and technology was needed in order to cope with the West. The shogunate, however, considered that this book censured its 200-year-long principle of isolation. Takano was arrested and after a long conflict with the government committed suicide. Siebold wrote the following about him:

> One of my efficient disciples, Takano Tsojoje from Ohosju, constantly accompanied me during 1826 until 1830. He helped me with Dutch translations from Japanese books and secretly travelled for me to the island of Tsushima and to the Japanese branch Busankai of Corea. When I left Japan, he wrote a booklet titled "Jume Monogatari" that describes his prophetic dream of a time when Japan abandoned its isolation. He also told me about scientific progress needed in his country and his own translations of useful European manuals. He seemed to me a strong, resolute, courageous young man[5].

Nevertheless, many Siebold disciples kept their faith in modern western sciences. This was the reason for Japan's speedy modernization during the Meji restoration.

So far we have discussed Siebold's contribution to Japan's social development. His political role has scarcely been considered before now. It is difficult to evaluate this adequately. I have been informed about some current research, but history reckons events by centuries, and that takes time, obviously.

[5] Diary of Philip Franz von Siebold 1859–1861 (travel reports in order of subjects) in: Toyo Bunko, archives of the parliamentary library of Tokyo.

Let us take for granted, however, Siebold's diplomatic activities between the 1930s and 1950s of his century. More and more important documents on his political activities have been found during recent years. We know about his influence on Dutch international politics, and his influence on Russian international politics is gradually being revealed[6]. In contrast to the United States and Great Britain, the Netherlands and Russia were trying to end Japan's politics of isolation peacefully. Both nations were trying to convince Japan to open up with mutual respect and estimation. Such a relationship was to be based on commercial exchange and profit. There is evidence, meanwhile, that Siebold himself intervened with the government authorities and not just with a cabinet member. Unfortunately, as we all know, the course of history was altered by the arrival of an American naval squadron in the Bay of Tokyo in 1853.

Anyhow, Siebold represented a highly appreciated idea of humanitarian concepts, in contrast to his contemporaries' opinions about underprivileged nations outside Europe.

The sympathetic reception Siebold received in Japan determined the image of Germany in Japan: the Japanese school system, the education of Japanese physicians and even army organization have all followed the German model. On the other hand, his extensive research entitles him to be considered as the founder of Japanese studies in Europe. It is fully justified to state that Siebold was a dominant influence in the formation of modern Japan. In his obituary of Siebold, Carl von Martius said in 1867 "Whatever an individual man, a scientist who even becomes diplomat, might be able to originate, he did it in word and writing".

[6] See Miyasaka M, Ishikawa M Neumann B (1994–1997) Siebold and Russia's policy of opening of Japan – a report on investigation of the Brandenstein-Zeppelin documents 1–3.In: Nanutaki Kiyo – Bulletin des Siebold Memorial Museums in Nagasaki, Nos. 4, 5, 7.

[7] Körner (1967), p. 923.

CHAPTER 9

The Activities of Philipp Franz von Siebold During His Second Stay in Japan, Particularly His Diplomatic Activities in Nagasaki, Yokohama and Edo

N. KUTSUZAWA

INTRODUCTION

In Japan as well as other countries many historical data have been kept about the activities of Siebold during his second visit to Japan. Studies of this topic, however, usually concentrate on the historical data available in each country separately. In this paper I am therefore going to use data from a wide range of countries. The material from Japan (see Table 1 for a more detailedlist) includes Bakumatsu Gaikoku Kankei Monjo, Zokutsushin Zenran, Oranda Shiiboruto Shoshin, Taiwasho, and Shiiboruto Kankei Shiryo; from Germany the diary of von Siebold (1861); from the Netherlands: Kolonien Geheim Verbaal and Dokumenten van het Nederlandse Consulaat Yokohama; and from Russia: Documents of the Central State Archive of the Navy (TSGAVMF). I want to use the above data comprehensively and will therefore concentrate on Siebold's diplomatic activities and make it clear to what extent he may have influenced the foreign policy of the Japanese Government.

PRELUDE TO SIEBOLD'S SECOND VISIT TO JAPAN

After returning to the Netherlands in 1829, Siebold did research based on the materials brought with him from Japan. He published the fruits of his research in the works *Nippon*, *Fauna Japonica*, *Flora Japonica*, etc., and with these achievements he became regarded as one of the three most famous European experts on Japan. The Dutch government tried to use his knowledge in its policies towards Japan. In 1844, the Dutch King Willem II asked Siebold to write a letter for him to the shogun of Japan with advice about the opening up of the country [1]. The

Table 1. Documents concerning the activities of Philipp Franz von Siebold during his second visit to Japan

Bakumatsu Gaikoku Kankei Monjo	Documents relating to foreign affairs during the Bakumatsu period (1853–1860)
Zoku Tsushin Zenran	Supplement to collection of diplomatic documents (1861–1868)
Oranda Shiiboruto Shoshin	Compilation of 11 letters in Dutch sent by Siebold between January 1861 and August 1866 to the Governor of Foreign Affairs and the Minister of Foreign Affairs
Taiwasho	Record of the conversations between Siebold and the Minister for Foreign Affairs, Ando Nobumasa, held on 10 June 1861
Shiiboruto Kankei Shiryo	Documents in Nagasaki relating to Siebold, compiled by Koga Jujiro
Diary of Siebold (1861)	Diary recording the activities of Siebold in the year 1861, written in German
Kolonien Geheim Verbaal	Compilation of documents sent to the Minister of Colonial Affairs of the Netherlands, including letters sent by Siebold to the minister relating his activities in Japan during 1859 and 1861
Dokumenten van het Nederlandse Consulaat Yokohama	Historical documents of the Dutch consulate in Yokohama, including letters sent by Siebold to the consulate in 1861
Documents of the Central State Archive of the Navy (TSGAVMF)	Documents in possession of the Russian Ministry for the Navy, including letters sent by Siebold to Admiral Lichacev between June and September 1861

letter strongly advised that it was dangerous to maintain old principles which forbade contacts between Japan and European countries. Siebold tried to spur the Dutch government to encourage the opening up of Japan by writing a draft treaty in 1852 called

"Siebold's draft treaty between the Netherlands or other countries and Japan" [2]. One of the main features of this proposal was that trade should be restricted to the harbor of Nagasaki. In 1853, Siebold wrote the "Draft treaty of commerce and navigation between Russia and Japan" (Entwurf eines Tractats für Schifffahren und Handelsverkehr von Seiten Russland mit Japan) (Fig. 1), which he showed not only to the Russian government but also to the Dutch Minister for Colonial Affairs. In a note attached to this treaty, Siebold mentions that the conclusion of this treaty by Russia and Japan would also lead to a new relationship between Russia and the Netherlands in Japan. This would serve the national interests of the Netherlands. He explained that profits could be made by bringing commodities from the Dutch Indies to Japan and delivering them to East Siberia and Kamchatka [3].

It is also widely known that Siebold asked to accompany the Japanese delegation to the American expedition squadron of Matthew Calbraith Perry, and that he advised the Russian government to include the demarcation of the frontier between Russia and Japan in negotiations with Japan. Eventually, he proposed that the Netherlands should set up an independent Japan Trading Company, and it was as an adviser to this Dutch company (Nederlandse Handelsmaatschappij) that he returned to Japan for the second time. In letters sent by Siebold to friends and acquaintances at the time of his departure, his reasons for going to Japan are expressed very clearly. In the first place he wanted to be of service to Japan. Another reason was a scientific one, namely the completion of his work *Nippon* [4]. So during his second stay in Japan Siebold became involved with Dutch policies towards Japan.

Siebold's Activities in Nagasaki

Siebold came back to Japan with his son Alexander on 4 August 1859 (Fig. 2) and presented a letter to the Governor of Nagasaki, Nagatsune Okabe (Fig. 3). He gave as a reason for his return to Japan that he wanted to play a role as a mediator between Japan and other countries, including the Netherlands [5]. Afterwards he continued to send letters to the Governor of Nagasaki and meet him regularly. At such meetings he made several suggestions about, for instance, the problem of currency exchange [6], bonded warehouses, the problem concerning the island of

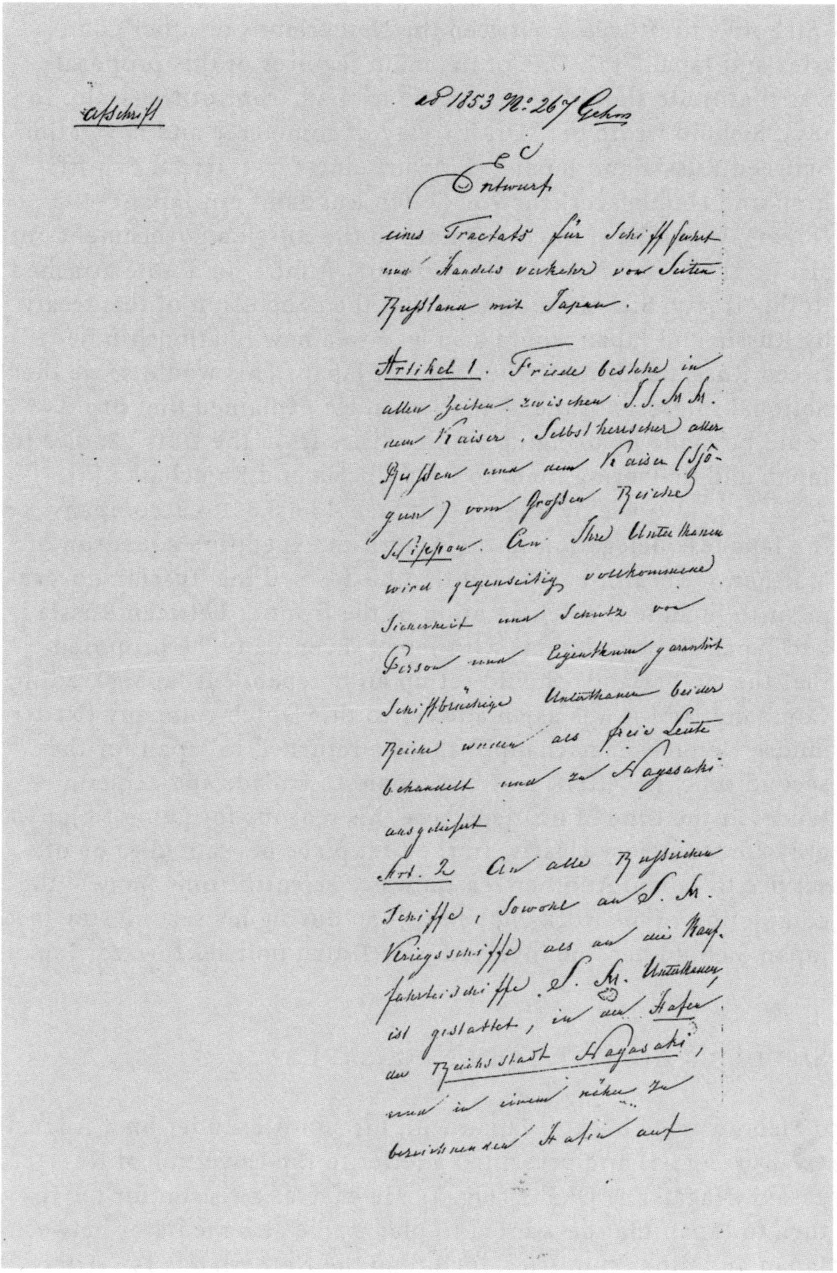
abschrift

ad 1853 No: 26 / Geheim

Entwurf

eines Tractats für Schifffahrt
und Handelsverkehr von Seiten
Russland mit Japan.

Artikel 1. Friede bestehe in
allen Zeiten zwischen S. S. M. M.
dem Kaiser, Selbstherrscher aller
Russen und dem Kaiser (Sjo-
gun) vom grossen Reiche
Nippon. An Ihre Unterthanen
wird gegenseitig vollkommene
Sicherheit und Schutz von
Person und Eigenthum garantirt
Schiffbrüchige Unterthanen beider
Reiche werden als freie Leute
behandelt und zu Nagasaki
ausgeliefert

Art. 2 An alle Russischen
Schiffe, sowohl an S. M.
Kriegsschiffe als an die Kauf-
fahrteischiffe S. M. Unterthanen
ist gestattet, in den Hafen
der Reichsstadt Nagasaki,
und in einem näher zu
bezeichnenden Hafen auf

Fig. 1. Draft of a treaty of commerce and navigation between Russia and Japan by Siebold. (National Archives, The Hague)

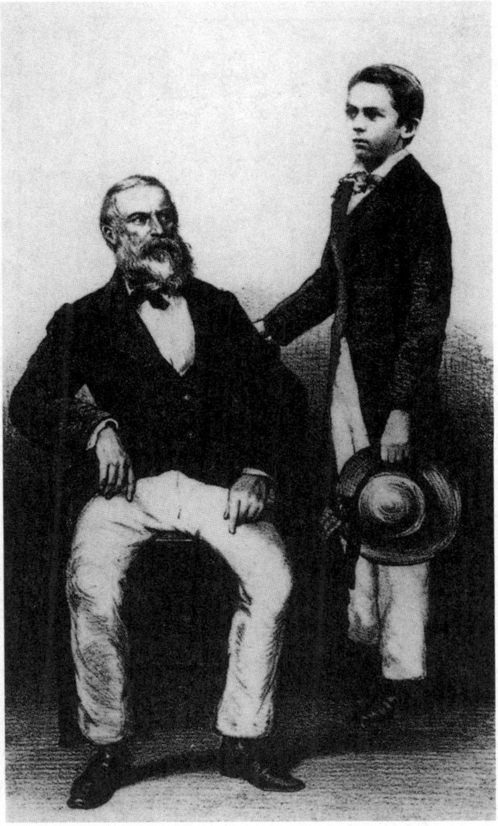

Fig. 2. Siebold and his son Alexander von Siebold. (Ph. F. von Siebold, Open brieven uit Japan, Dejima 1861)

Tsushima [7], and the plan to open the harbor of Nagasaki as a free port for foreign ships [8].

Regarding the Tsushima problem , Siebold strongly advised Japan not to grant England and France, which had become more interested in Japan after the Arrow incident, land on this island to use as a naval port. Nevertheless, to prevent future trouble both countries should be offered a section of the harbor of Tsushima. Siebold also expressed his discontent with the practice of currency exchange whereby Japan was obliged to offer a fixed amount of Japanese silver coins; according to him this practice was clearly advantageous to foreign countries. These activities of Siebold meant that he became known in the capital, Edo, and eventually the Japanese Government invited him to come to Yokohama for consultation on scientific and other matters [9].

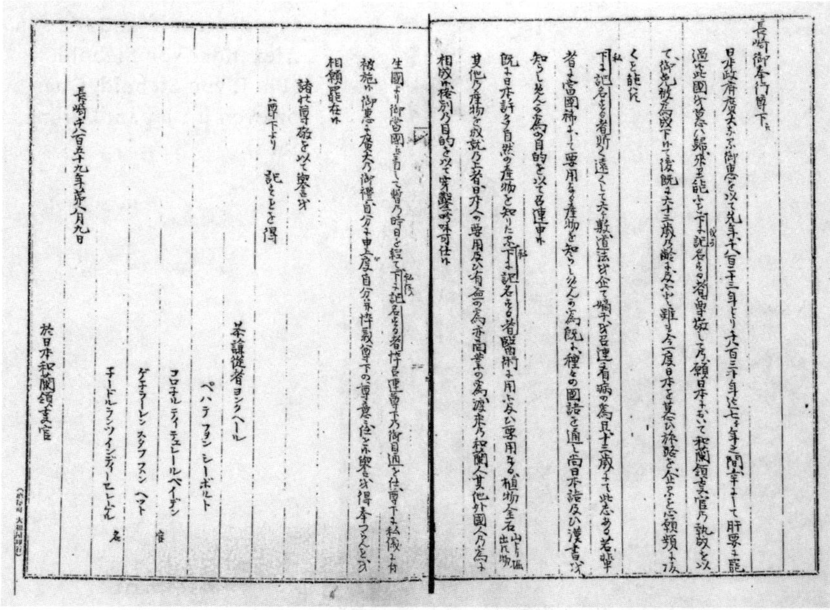
長崎御奉行閣下

相願罷在候

恭謙従者ヨンクヘール
ペハテ フヲン シーボルト

長崎千八百五十九年第八月九日

於日本和蘭領事官

Fig. 3. Siebold's letter to the governor of Nagasaki (in Japanese). (Nagasaki prefectural library, Nagasaki)

SIEBOLD'S ACTIVITIES IN YOKOHAMA

Siebold and his son Alexander arrived in Yokohama on 4 April 1861 and met the Governor of Kanagawa, Yasunao Matsudaira (Fig. 4). This governor asked Siebold various questions about the general situation in the countries Japan had concluded treaties with, about the basic policy line of the Japanese mission to Europe, and about the possibility of moving the trade harbor from Yokohama to another port. Siebold answered those questions as follows. First he described the state of affairs in various countries. Concerning England he explained that it was the factory of the world and in order to sell its manufacturing products was constantly opening up new markets. There was the possibility that England would start a conflict if its intentions were hindered. It was therefore necessary to be cautious with England, but also with countries like America and France. On the other hand, Siebold thought that Russia needed Japan to provide many commodities for the Russians living in the northern part of east-

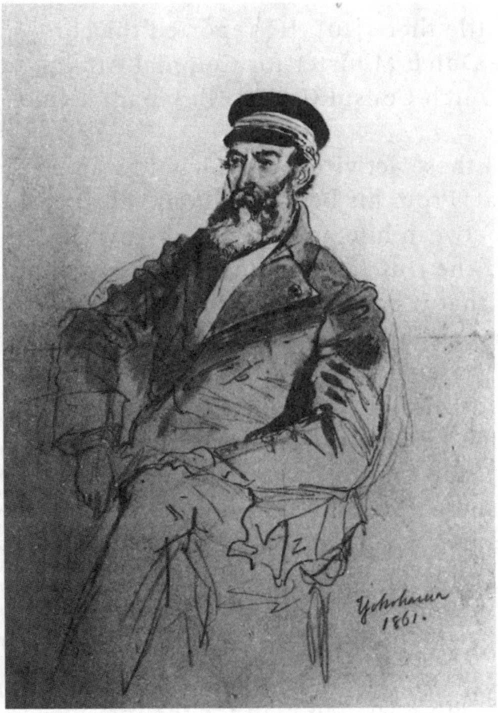

Fig. 4. Portrait of Siebold, sketched by Charles Wirgman in Yokohama [4]

ern Asia, and was in need of a harbor and supply base in Japan for its navy. He also believed that Russia did not intend to invade Japan. Siebold regarded the Prussian army as very strong and stressed the importance of good relations with that country. He gave some accounts of Holland and Portugal, but for some reason he didn't say much about the importance of the relationship between Japan and Holland.

Furthermore, Siebold advised the Governor that the mission sent to Europe should pay special attention to the army, the navy, and the army schools. He mentioned that the success of this mission would be crucial for Japan to keep its peace and prosperity for the coming decade. He also proposed that Nagasaki should be opened as a free port for foreign ships, and that bonded warehouses should be built there. He thought it possible to move the trading port to Nagasaki, because if docks were built in Akunoura and Nagasaki became an important trading place for Japanese products, then it would also become attractive enough for merchants to settle there [10]. He reported the contents of this meeting to the Dutch Minister for Colonial Affairs, James Loudon, and to the Dutch Consul General in Japan, J.K. de Wit [11].

One can discern from these activities that Siebold wanted to become a Dutch diplomat. From his behavior, however, it is clear that there was a gap between him and the Dutch government. Namely, the policy of the Dutch government at this period had changed in such a way that it cooperated with other countries in demanding from Japan that all the ports should be

opened as agreed since the Ansei Treaty. Siebold, however, believed in pressing for just one harbor to be opened, in Nagasaki, and he was trying to push the Japanese government in that direction. It was this point that made the Dutch government decide that it had to show the Japanese government, from the viewpoint of foreign policy towards Japan, what the relationship with Siebold was. Siebold was also trying to make a good impression on the Russians by reporting the contents of this meeting in a letter to the Russian commander of the Eastern Fleet, Ivan Feodoric Lichacev [12]. After that, he presented the Minister for Foreign Affairs, Takeuchi Yasunori, with a written plan for the mission. Siebold stated in that plan that he wanted to join the mission and would like to offer his services. He also advised that the mission to Europe should pay especially close attention to military science, navigation, shipbuilding, mining, machinery and agriculture, and recommended that they should study those areas and adopt any useful aspects [13]. We can again very clearly see here Siebold's approach of trying to build a bridge between Japan and other countries.

Siebold's Activities in Edo

On 18 June 1861 Siebold and Alexander arrived in Edo (Fig. 5) at the Akabane House where the Prussian ambassador was living [14]. There he was asked by the Governors for Foreign Affairs, Torii Tadayoshi and Tsuda Masamichi, to provide some scientific training for medical doctors and academic scholars. But Siebold stressed that he wanted to give advice on more pressing matters such as foreign relations or trade rather than on medicine or other sciences [15]. Although officially the Japanese gov-

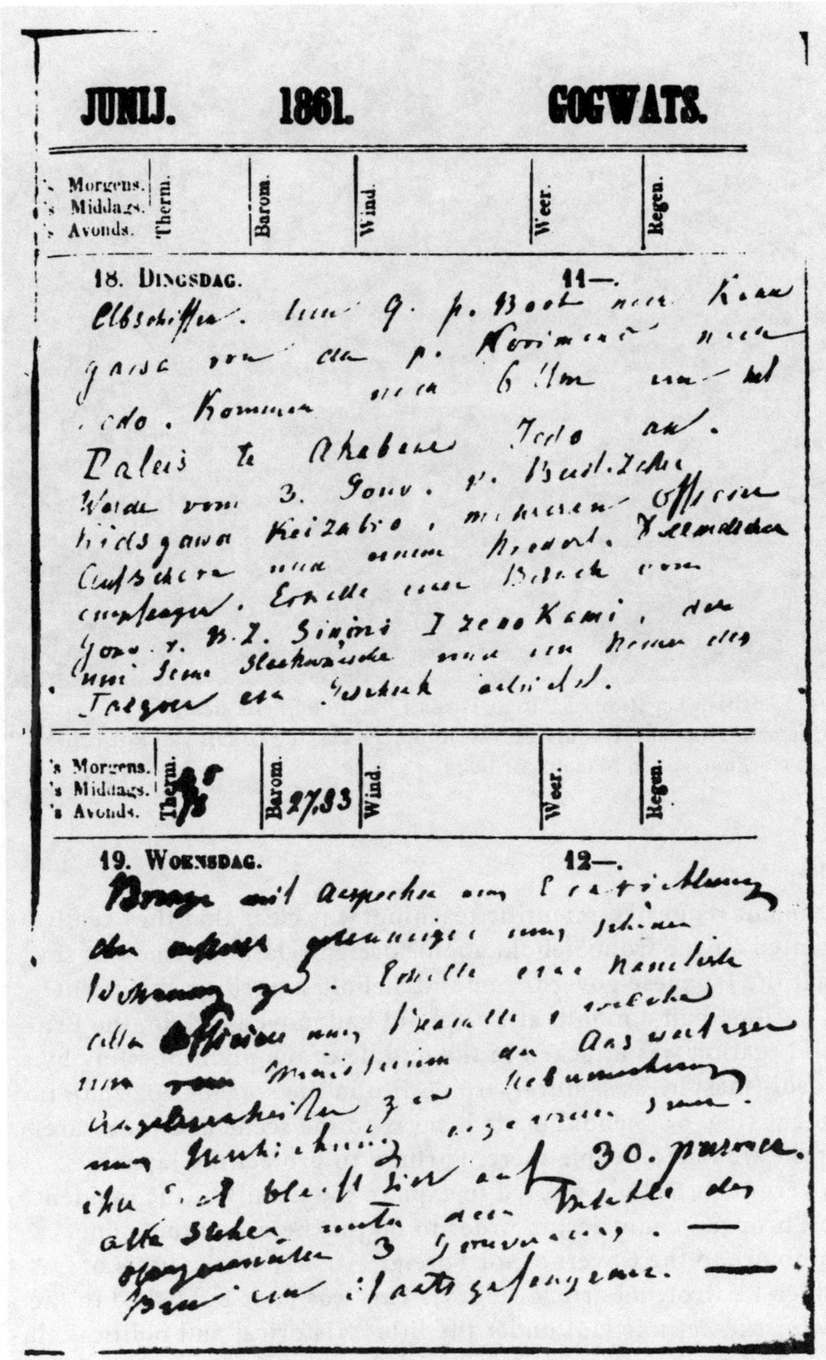

Fig. 5. Siebold's diary of 1861. (Nagasaki prefectural library, Nagasaki)

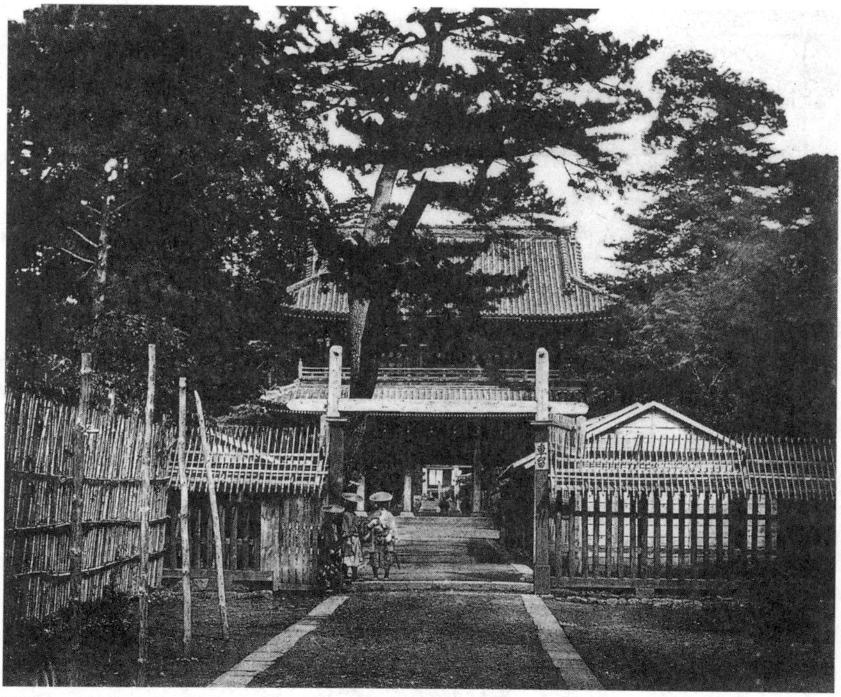

Fig. 6. British Legation of Edo in Tozenji. Photo by Felix Beato (Herman J. Moeshart, Journaal van Jonkheer Dirk de Graeff van Polsbroek, Van Gorgum, Assen Maastricht,1987)

ernment requested scientific teaching, it is clear that they really wanted advice from Siebold about foreign relations. One can say that the Japanese government and Siebold agreed on this point.

Just half a month after Siebold had moved to Edo, the British Legation was attacked in the middle of the night of 5 July by a Roshi (masterless samurai) from Mito in the so-called Tozenji incident (Fig. 6). Siebold made his way to the scene and took care of the wounded people there. Further, to protect the Japanese government Siebold wanted to explain the details of the incident to European countries; in order to do this he presented a questionnaire to the Governor for Foreign Affairs, on the basis of which he wrote an article (Fig. 7). This was later published in the *Kölnische Zeitung* [16] under the title "Historical and political elucidation on the attack on the British Legation in Tozenji Temple at Edo" [17] (Fig. 8).

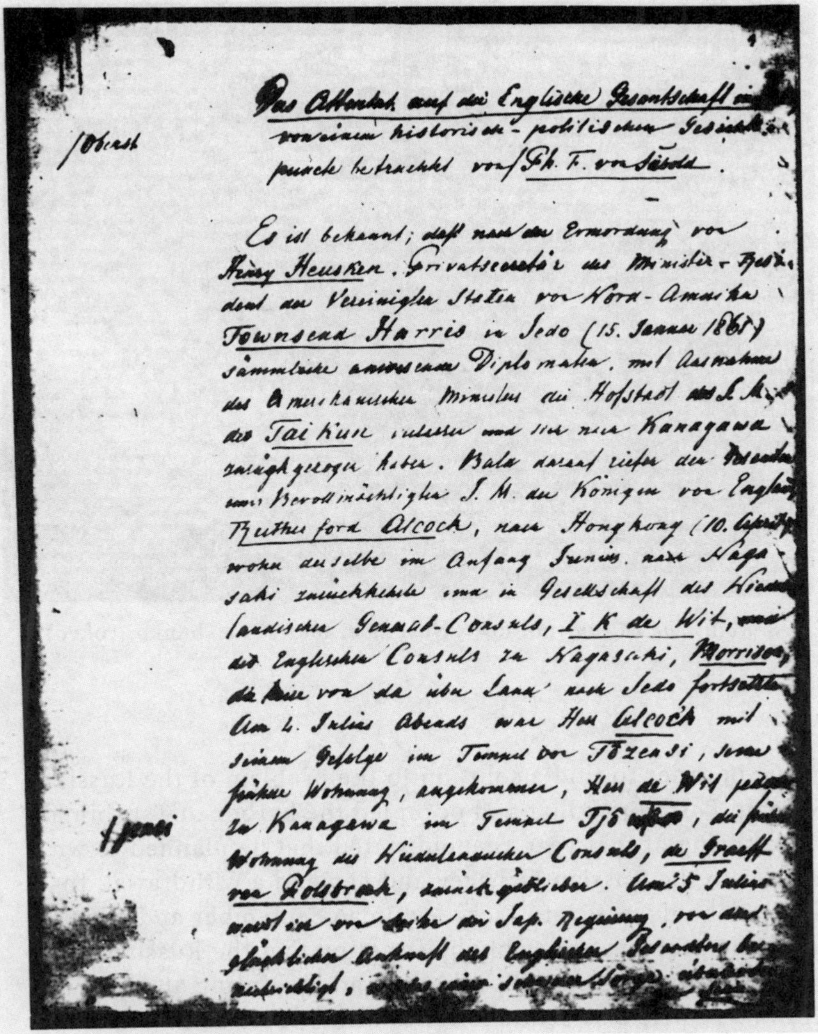

Das Attentat auf die Englische Gesandtschaft in [illegible]
von einem historisch-politischen Gesichts-
punkte betrachtet von Ph. F. von Siebold.

Es ist bekannt; daß nach der Ermordung von
Henry Heusken, Privatsecretär des Minister-Resi-
denten der Vereinigten Staaten von Nord-Amerika
Townsend Harris in Jedo (15. Januar 1861)
sämmtliche anwesenden Diplomaten, mit Ausnahme
des Amerikanischen Ministers die Hofstadt des S. M.
des Taikun verlassen und sich nach Kanagawa
zurückgezogen haben. Bald darauf reiste der Gesandte
und Bevollmächtigte I. M. der Königin von England
Rutherford Alcock, nach Hongkong (10. April)
wohin derselbe im Anfang Junius nach Naga-
saki zurückkehrte und in Gesellschaft des Nieder-
ländischen General-Consuls, I K de Wit, und
des Englischen Consuls zu Nagasaki, Morrison,
die Reise von da über Land nach Jedo fortsetzte.
Am 4. Julius Abends war Herr Alcock mit
seinem Gefolge im Tempel von Tôzensi, seiner
früheren Wohnung, angekommen, Herr de Wit jedoch
zu Kanagawa im Tempel Tjô [illegible], die frühere
Wohnung des Niederländischen Consuls, de Graeff
van Polsbroek, zurückgeblieben. Am 5. Julius
wurde er von Seiten der Jap. Regierung von der
glücklichen Ankunft des Englischen Gesandten be-
nachrichtigt, [illegible]

Fig. 7. Article by Siebold about the Tozenji Incident. (Toyo bunko, Tokyo)

During the meeting held at the house of Nobumasa Ando, the Minister of Foreign Affairs, immediately after the Tozenji Incident, Siebold proposed that the opening of the harbor of Nagasaki as a free port for foreign ships should be a negotiating point for the Japanese mission to Europe. Siebold said that he could solve this problem by joining the mission and negotiating directly with the heads of state of each country [18]. Further-

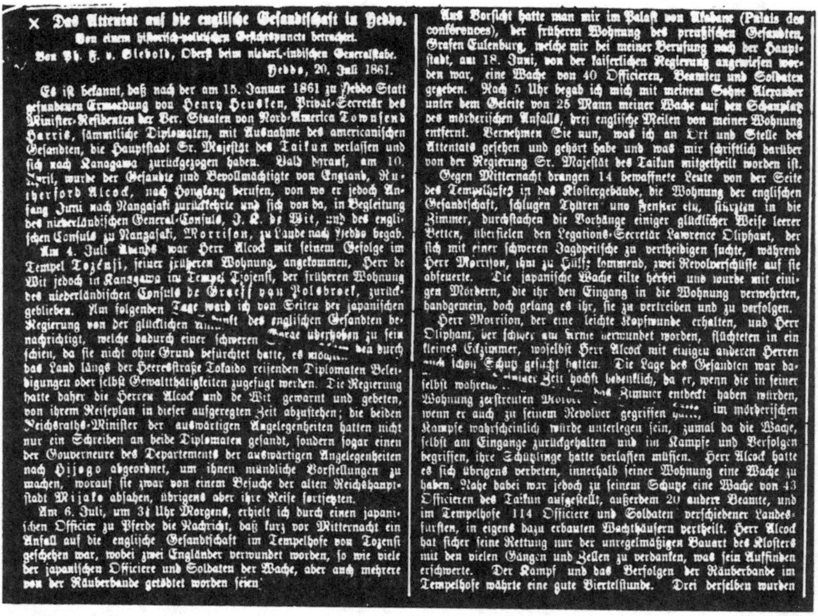

× Das Attentat auf die englische Gesandtschaft in Yeddo.

Von einem historisch-politischen Gesichtspuncte betrachtet.

Von Ph. F. v. Siebold, Oberst beim niederl.-indischen Generalstabe.

Yeddo, 20. Juli 1861.

Es ist bekannt, daß nach der am 15. Januar 1861 zu Yeddo Statt gefundenen Ermordung von Henry Heusken, Privat-Secretär des Minister-Residenten der Ver. Staaten von Nord-America Townsend Harris, sämmtliche Diplomaten, mit Ausnahme des americanischen Gesandten, die Hauptstadt Sr. Majestät des Taikun verlassen und sich nach Kanagawa zurückgezogen haben. Bald darauf, am 10. April, wurde der Gesandte und Bevollmächtigte von England, Rutherford Alcock, nach Hongkong berufen, von wo er jedoch Anfang Juni nach Nangasaki zurückkehrte und sich von da, in Begleitung des niederländischen General-Consuls, J. K. de Wit, und des englischen Consuls zu Nangasaki, Morrison, zu Lande nach Yeddo begab.

Am 4. Juli Abends war Herr Alcock mit seinem Gefolge im Tempel Tozensi, seiner früheren Wohnung, angekommen, Herr de Wit jedoch in Kanagawa im Tempel Tiojensi, der früheren Wohnung des niederländischen Consuls de Graeff van Polsbroek, zurückgeblieben. Am folgenden Tage ward ich von Seiten der japanischen Regierung von der glücklichen An[illegible]nft des englischen Gesandten benachrichtigt, welche dadurch einer schweren [illegible]rge überhoben zu sein schien, da sie nicht ohne Grund befürchtet hatte, es möch[illegible] den durch das Land längs der Heerstraße Tokaido reisenden Diplomaten Beleidigungen oder selbst Gewaltthätigkeiten zugefugt werden. Die Regierung hatte daher die Herren Alcock und de Wit gewarnt und gebeten, von ihrem Reiseplan in dieser aufgeregten Zeit abzustehen; die beiden Reichsraths-Minister der auswärtigen Angelegenheiten hatten nicht nur ein Schreiben an beide Diplomaten gesandt, sondern sogar einen der Gouverneure des Departements der auswärtigen Angelegenheiten nach Hijogo abgeordnet, um ihnen mündliche Vorstellungen zu machen, worauf sie zwar von einem Besuche der alten Reichshauptstadt Mijako absahen, übrigens aber ihre Reise fortsetzten.

Am 6. Juli, um 3½ Uhr Morgens, erhielt ich durch einen japanischen Officier zu Pferde die Nachricht, daß kurz vor Mitternacht ein Anfall auf die englische Gesandtschaft im Tempelhofe von Tozensi geschehen war, wobei zwei Engländer verwundet worden, so wie viele der japanischen Officiere und Soldaten der Wache, aber auch mehrere von der Räuberbande getödtet worden seien.

Aus Vorsicht hatte man mir im Palast von Akabane (Palais des conférences), der früheren Wohnung des preußischen Gesandten, Grafen Eulenburg, welche mir bei meiner Berufung nach der Hauptstadt, am 18. Juni, von der kaiserlichen Regierung angewiesen worden war, eine Wache von 40 Officieren, Beamten und Soldaten gegeben. Nach 5 Uhr begab ich mich mit meinem Sohne Alexander unter dem Geleite von 25 Mann meiner Wache auf den Schauplatz des mörderischen Anfalls, drei englische Meilen von meiner Wohnung entfernt. Vernehmen Sie nun, was ich an Ort und Stelle des Attentats gesehen und gehört habe und was mir schriftlich darüber von der Regierung Sr. Majestät des Taikun mitgetheilt worden ist.

Gegen Mitternacht drangen 14 bewaffnete Leute von der Seite des Tempelhofes in das Klostergebäude, die Wohnung der englischen Gesandtschaft, schlugen Thüren und Fenster ein, stürzten in die Zimmer, durchstachen die Vorhänge einiger glücklicher Weise leerer Betten, überfielen den Legations-Secretär Lawrence Oliphant, der sich mit einer schweren Jagdpeitsche zu vertheidigen suchte, während Herr Morrison, ihm zu Hülfe kommend, zwei Revolverschüsse auf sie abfeuerte. Die japanische Wache eilte herbei und wurde mit einigen Mördern, die ihr den Eingang in die Wohnung verwehrten, handgemein, doch gelang es ihr, sie zu vertreiben und zu verfolgen.

Herr Morrison, der eine leichte Kopfwunde erhalten, und Herr Oliphant, der schwer am Arme verwundet worden, flüchteten in ein kleines Eckzimmer, woselbst Herr Alcock mit einigen anderen Herren auch schon Schutz gesucht hatten. Die Lage des Gesandten war daselbst während [illegible] Zeit höchst bedenklich, da er, wenn die in seiner Wohnung zerstreuten Mörder [illegible] das Zimmer entdeckt haben würden, wenn er auch zu seinem Revolver gegriffen hätte, im mörderischen Kampfe wahrscheinlich würde unterlegen sein, zumal da die Wache, selbst am Eingange zurückgehalten und im Kampfe und Verfolgen begriffen, ihre Schützlinge hatte verlassen müssen. Herr Alcock hatte es sich übrigens verbeten, innerhalb seiner Wohnung eine Wache zu haben. Nahe dabei war jedoch zu seinem Schutze eine Wache von 43 Officieren des Taikun aufgestellt, außerdem 20 andere Beamte, und im Tempelhofe 114 Officiere und Soldaten verschiedener Landesfürsten, in eigens dazu erbauten Wachthäusern vertheilt. Herr Alcock hat sicher seine Rettung nur der unregelmäßigen Bauart des Klosters mit den vielen Gängen und Zellen zu verdanken, was sein Auffinden erschwerte. Der Kampf und das Verfolgen der Räuberbande im Tempelhofe währte eine gute Viertelstunde. Drei derselben wurden

Fig. 8. *Kölnische Zeitung* no. 307, 5 November 1861. (Toyo bunko, Tokyo)

more, in order to find a solution to the problem of the Russian warship *Possadnick* that had occupied the harbor of Tsushima since spring of that year, Siebold stated that he planned to write a letter to the Russian Lichacev and demand a withdrawal. Indeed, Siebold wrote a to Lichacev on 26 September and tried to solve the problem peaceably by stressing that the Russian settlement on Tsushima raised problems and by hinting at a withdrawal [19]. He also sent a letter to Minister Ando in which he tried to provide a solution for handling the Tozenji incident. In order to win back the trust of foreign countries, he suggested the following [20]:

- According to international law a legation was a place not to be trespassed on; violation of this law or an attack on such a place was therefore a grave offense and should be punished severely.
- If the government did not take severe measures it was not unthinkable that the incident would escalate into war.

- The government must arrest the perpetrator and make clear what the reasons were for this attack on the legation.

The details of the conversations during this meeting were recorded in Taiwasho.

Siebold informed the Dutch Minister for Colonial Affairs and Lichacev from Russia about the Tozenji incident [21]. After that, important talks were held between the Japanese government and Alcock in Ando'shouse on 14 and 15 August. During these meetings Alcock demanded guarantees that the items for negotiation put on the agenda by the Japanese mission could only include the opening of the cities of Edo and Osaka and the ports of Hyogo and Niigata to free trade by foreigners. The Japanese government agreed with this demand [22] (Fig. 9). One can see this as a change in the foreign policy of the Japanese government, which now tried to use Britain's power to solve the problems with Russia regarding Tsushima. Moreover, there were complaints from de Wit about Siebold's behavior in Edo, where he acted like a diplomat but was not officially one. For these reasons, the Japanese government eventually made it clear to Siebold that his scientific work was to be suspended [23]. This meant that he was also dismissed as a diplomatic adviser. So ended Siebold's second visit to Japan, in just two and a half years.

Nevertheless, we can see distinctly in Siebold's approach and activities during the Tozenji incident, especially from his article in *Kölnische Zeitung*, that he tried to be a mediator between Japan and other countries. His advice that the Japanese mission to Europe should have a close look at the countries visited and adopt the elements that would be useful for Japan did not find a willing ear among Japanese government officials at that time. In the Meiji period, however, one member of the mission, Terajima Munenori, applied Siebold's advice by establishing a telegraph service. One can see this as a fulfillment of Siebold's proposals [24].

Conclusion

From the above we can conclude the following. The activities of Siebold during his second stay in Japan had a strong politi-

leur assurerait des résultats incalculables de grandeur; ces mêmes hommes, supposant le fait accompli, mettent en doute que les Puissances Alliées puissent, sans sacrifices immenses, arrêter le développement de la Puissance subitement gigantesque, devenue le lot des Czars dans l'extrême Asie. * * * *

La Corée est divisée en deux partis politiques.

Tout ce qui a été dit et écrit sur les richesses aurifères de la Californie n'est rien auprès de ce qui a été rapporté de celles de la Corée, pays qui est aussi excessivement riche en cuivre. L'or y est si abondant qu'il est défendu, sous peine de mort, de la ramasser, pour ne pas trop avilir le numéraire en circulation.

No. 10.

Mr. Alcock to Lord J. Russell.—(Received October 28.)

114 (Confidential.)

My Lord,

Yeddo, August 16, 1861.

IN my despatch of the 2nd instant I submitted to your Lordship all the information attainable here on the subject of Russian designs in the Japanese seas. I propose now to bring under notice the present state of our relations, and those of other Treaty Powers in this country, with especial reference to your despatch No. 43 of the 10th of April last, respecting the opening of Yeddo as a place of residence for British subjects on the 1st of January next; and also to a letter addressed by the Tycoon to Her Majesty, and another from the Ministers of Foreign Affairs to myself, translations of which are inclosed. The purport of both is to urge the expediency, if not the necessity, of deferring for a period of seven years the opening of Yeddo to foreigners generally, and the other ports designated in the Treaty.

The attack on the Legation, and this proposition of the Japanese Government to defer the execution of Treaties in regard to the opening of new ports for trade, and any additional points of contact with the people, are simultaneous events of great significance and importance. Coming together they seem to point with no doubtful meaning to a crisis in our relations. It is, indeed, impossible not to feel, here on the spot, that we have arrived at a turning-point in the history of all foreign relations with Japan, or to doubt that on the course now taken by both Contracting Parties will greatly depend what shall be the final issue of the efforts hitherto made by Treaty and Resident Ministers at the capital to establish on a permanent basis of goodwill and mutual advantage political and commercial relations with a country so long and so obstinately persisting in a policy of isolation.

In proportion to the importance of this issue is the responsibility grave which attaches to the action of the foreign Representatives now in Yeddo. A false step on their part at so critical a moment might plunge the country into a civil war, or equally throw everything into confusion, under the alarm and excitement of any anticipations of foreign war. Error even in another direction, by excess of caution, may give such encouragement to the hostile agencies at work, that the position created by Treaties will be too far lost to be ever recovered by peaceable means.

Your Lordship will readily conceive my anxiety to avoid both these dangers, the Scylla and Charybdis of the actual situation; and that it has required wary steering not to be influenced by fanciful dangers nor paralysed by those which were only too real, with all the consciousness that too much caution would be at least as fatal as rashness or boldness in the wrong place.

After more than a month thus passed, I hope I can now give your Lordship such assurances of success in this perilous navigation as shall relieve Her Majesty's Government of much immediate anxiety, give them the necessary time to come to a deliberate opinion as to the policy they will adopt, and better hope, withal, of final good resulting than has hitherto appeared warranted.

I could not have said so much a week ago; but yesterday brought a new phase, and will, in all probability, be seen hereafter to make an epoch in the history of our relations. The object of two years' labour and seemingly fruitless effort was gained, and the want of which had always been felt fatal to any steady or sure progress with Japanese rulers. I succeeded in obtaining what I had well nigh despaired of, a confidential interview with the Foreign Ministers, to the exclusion of the Governors of Foreign Affairs, all subordinate officers, and attendants of every class. And the result of this first commencement of really confidential relations will, I feel satisfied, not only be felt in present benefit, but prove, long years hence, to be the very pivot on which will turn the whole character of the future intercourse between foreigners and Japanese.

I went on the 14th instant to present Admiral Hope, who had landed the day before,

cal and diplomatic content. One can see this as an extension of the letter to the shogun that he was asked to write by King Willem II and which contained advice about the opening up of Japan. From the fact that he sent notes of his activities in Japan to the Dutch Minister for Colonial Affairs and the Dutch Consul General in Japan, we can see that he was not only trying to improve his reputation further but that he also wished to be appointed as a Dutch diplomatic representative in Japan.

The basic attitude of Siebold was that he would agree to work for the country that acknowledged his intellectual competence and knowledge and the fact that he was a source of information about Japan.

At first he worked for the Netherlands; after his return to Europe he was approached by Russia and France. In 1865 he proposed to Emperor Napoleon III that a Franco-Japanese Trading Company should be set up [25]. One can suppose that this was because the French evaluated Siebold's knowledge of Japan positively.

Besides Siebold's diplomatic activities during his second visit to Japan, he was also occupied with a wide range of academic activities such as scientific lectures [26], completing his research work *Nippon* [27], writing a continuation of his work *Flora Japonica* [28], compiling a Japanese-Dutch-English-French Dictionary [29], and collecting ethnologic material [30]. Indeed, one can say that Siebold'g second stay in Japan had various objects, making his activities very diverse.

References

1. Chijs JA van der (1867) Neerlands sterven tot openstelling van Japan voor den Wereldhandel. Frederik Muller, Amsterdam, pp 47—52
2. Chijs JA van der (1867) Neerlands sterven tot openstelling van Japan voor den Wereldhandel. Frederik Muller, Amsterdam, pp 79—85
3. Algemeen Rijksarchief, Minister van Kolonien (National Archives, The Hague), Geheim Verbaal no. 5841, August 22, 1853, no. 312

←

Fig. 9. Alcock's letter to Lord Russell, 16 August 1861. (In Confidential Paper relating to Affairs in Japan Fo410—3, Yokohama Archives of History, Yokkohama)

4. Körner H (1967) Die Würzburger Siebold. Eine Gelehrten Familie des 18. und 19. Jahrhundert. Barth, Leipzig, pp 448—453
5. Shiiboruto Kankei Shiryo, p 10 (Nagasaki Prefectural Library Nagasaki) (in Japanese)
6. Bakumatsu Gaikoku Kankei Monjo 36, Tokyo Daigaku Shuppankai, 1986, p 184 (in Japanese)
7. Bakumatsu Gaikoku Kankei Monjo 42, Tokyo Daigaku Shuppankai, 1989, pp 256—257 (in Japanese)
8. Maclean J (1978) Philipp Franz von Siebold and opening of Japan 1843—1860. In: Philipp Franz von Siebold: a contribution to the study of historical relations between Japan and the Netherlands. The Netherlands Association for Japanese Studies, p 71

9. Zoku Tsushin Zenran, Hennen no. Bu 2, Bunkyu Gannen (1861), Yushodo Shuppan, 1983, p 62 (in Japanese)
10. Algemeen Rijksarchief, Minister van Kolonien (National Archives, The Hague), Geheim Verbaal no. 5923, May 7, 1863 no. 94 Bijlage M, Bijlage N
11. Algemeen Rijksarchief, Consulaat Yokohama (National Archives, The Hague), Algemeen Correspondence 4 1861 August—December, Afschrift Bijlage L.A Geheim 23 April 1861
12. Siebold's letter to Lichacev, May 17. 1861. In: Koichi Yasuda (ed) Bunkyu Gannen no Tairo Gaiko to Shiiboruto. Okayamadaigaku Kibi Yogakushiryo kenkyukai 1995, pp 120—122
13. Zoku Tsushin Zenran, Hennen no Bu 2, Bunkyu Gannen (1861), Yushodo Shuppan, 1983: pp 59—62 (in Japanese)
14. Diary of Siebold in 1861 (photostat in Toyobunko, Tokyo)
15. Zoku Tsushin Zenran, Hennen no Bu 2, Bunkyu Gannen (1861), Yushodo Shuppan, 1983, pp 86 (in Japanese)
16. Kölnishe Zeitung, no. 307, November 5, 1861, Das Attentat auf die englische Gesandtschaft in Edo vom einem historische-politischen Gesichtspunkt betrachtet
17. Nobukata Kutsuzawa. Tozenji Jiken ni Miru Shiiboruto no Gaikoteki Katsudo ni tsuite, Kenji Yanai (ed) Yoshikawa Kobunkan, 1988 (in Japanese)
18. Taiwasho. In: Koichi Yasuda (ed) Bunkyu Gannnen no Tairo Gaiko to Shiiboruto, Okayamadaigaku Kibi Yogakushiryo kenkyukai 1995, p 230 (in Japanese)
19. Siebold's letter to Lichacev, September 26. 1861. In: Koichi Yasuda (ed) Bunkyu Gannen no Tairo Gaiko to Shiiboruto. Okayamadaigaku Kibi Yogakushiryo kenkyukai 1995, pp 129—131
20. Maclean J (1978) Philipp Franz von Siebold and opening of Japan 1843—1860. In: Philipp Franz von Siebold: a contribution to the study of historical relations between Japan and the Netherlands. The Netherlands Association for Japanese Studies, p 77
21. Algemeen Rijksarchief, Minister van Kolonien (National Archives, The Hague), Geheim Verbaal no. 5923 May 1863, 94 (Bijlage U)

22. Alcock's letter to Lord J. Russell, August 16. 1861, In: Confidential paper relating to affairs in Japan, F.o.410—3, pp 44 (Photo Yokohama Archives of History, Yokohama)
23. Zoku Tsushin Zenran, Hennen no Bu 2, Bunkyu Gannen (1861), Yushodo Shuppan, 1983, p 174 (in Japanese)
24. Nobukata Kutsuzawa. Takeuchi Shisetsudan to Seiyobunmei-Denshin donyu wo chushin ni. In: Yogaku Kotohajime Bakumatsu Meijishoki ni okeru Seiyobunmei no Donyu ni kansuru Kenkyukai (ed.) Bunkashobo Hakubunsha 1993, pp 223—245 (in Japanese)
25. Körner H (1967) Die Würzburger Siebold. Eine Gelehrten Familie des 18. und 19. Jahrhundert. Barth, Leipzig, p 472
26. Algemeen Rijksarchief, Minister van Kolonien (National Archives, The Hague), Geheim Verbaal no.5923 May 7.1863, no.94 Bijlage DD
27. Mise Morobuchi Sensei Ihinbunken Mokuroku, Matuyama Kotoshogyo Gakko Shoji Chosakai 1937, p 9 (in Japanese)
28. Yoshikazu Ishiyama. 1864nen Würzburg kara no Kokaijo, In: Seibutsugakushi Kenkyu no. 46, 1985, p 26 (in Japanese)
29. Siebold's letter to Roju, January 10. 1861, In: Oranda Shiiboruto Shoshin (Historiographical Institute, The University of Tokyo, Tokyo)
30. Algemeen Rijksarchief, Consulaat Yokohama (National Archives, The Hague), Algemeen Correspondence 3, 1861 January—July Nagasaki, no. 117 March 28, 1861

CHAPTER 10

Siebold the Research Manager*

H. Beukers

Imagine the following job description: "Wanted, a person willing to gather and publish detailed information about the geography, natural history, arts and sciences, religions, mythology, folk culture, history, natural resources, trade and public institutions of a country named Nippon. The country extends between latitude 46° and 24° N and is at a rough estimate 370,000 km^2 (which is about ten times the size of the Netherlands). The country is not accessible to foreigners, with the exception of Chinese and Dutch traders, who are confined to isolated areas in the harbor of Nagasaki, in the country's south-western part, far from the seat of the government in Edo. Only the captain, the head of the Dutch settlement at Dejima, and two assistants are allowed to make a quadrennial visit to Edo, the so-called court-journey."

The Dutch government could have described in this way the position of the key figure in the restoration and enlargement of commerce with Japan after the Napoleonic wars and the British occupation of the Dutch colonies in Asia.

Baron van der Capellen, the governor-general of the Dutch East Indies, who gave shape to that policy regarding commerce, refined the requirements for the position. Taking into account the restrictions on contact between the Dutch and the inhabitants of Nagasaki, he thought that inquiries as described could only be made by an official who enjoyed the confidence of those inhabitants. In this respect he considered the doctor on the island of Dejima was crucial. There was great interest in western medical sciences in Japan. A learned and successful physician with wide interests could build up the necessary relationships, particularly

* Presented at the Siebold Memorial International Medical Symposium, Huis ten Bosch, 28 September 1996.

with the *Rangakusha,* Japanese scholars who were interested in "Dutch" sciences.

In modem terms, we would define the position as research manager. The person to be appointed would be in charge of a gigantic research project which needed accurate planning and coordination and the support and cooperation of many people, not just during field research when a great variety of items and data would be collected but also in the working up of the collected material and the final publication of the results.

Once Govemor-General van der Capellen had met the young Bavarian physician Philipp Franz von Siebold in 1823, he was convinced that this was the right man for the special mission. What convinced the Govemor-General? Probably not Siebold's medical experience. After graduation in 1820, he had practiced medicine for only 2 years before he decided to leave for the Dutch East Indies. Apart from many excellent recommendations from eminent German scholars, it must have been Siebold's background. Philipp Franz was by descent predestined to become medical doctor. His grandfather, father and uncles constituted the so-called Academia Sieboldiana, the famous medical faculty of Würzburg at the turn of the eighteenth century. Their successors gave the young Siebold a thorough and up-to-date medical education.

Grandfather Carl Caspar Siebold established one of the Leiden–Wiirzburg connections. During his study tour in the 1760s, he followed, among others, the courses of the anatomist Albinus and the clinician Gaubius in Leiden. His visit to the successors of the famous medical teacher Herman Boerhaave was in line with the developments in medical teaching in Würzburg after the reformation by Karl Philipp von Greiffenklau in 1749, when the curriculum became strongly influenced by Boerhaave and his pupils. Following the Boerhaavian model, the curriculum was based on the natural sciences and had a strong practical orientation. This positivist, anti-speculative tendency was still dominant during Philipp Franz's years of study. The Würzburg clinic was for instance under the supervision of the famous Johann Lucas von Schoenlein, who argued for genuine empirical methods to be used in internal medicine, analogous to those used in natural history. These methods consisted of accurate observations, descriptions and comparisons, independent of theoretical speculations. That rational-empirical attitude dominated Siebold's medical education.

Siebold's broader scientific training was strongly determined by the Würzburg professor of anatomy and physiology, Ignaz Döllinger, friend of Siebold's father since his youth. Döllinger was prominent in basic medical sciences and well versed in botany. Philipp Franz stayed in Döllinger's house during his student days. Here he studied anatomy and botany almost daily under his host's supervision. The house was also a meeting-place for prominent scientists such as the brothers Nees von Esenbeck, both eminent botanists. In this stimulating scientific environment the young student developed a lifelong liking for natural history. Siebold's desire to study the natural history of other continents dated from that period. It was this interest that prompted him to join an expedition to Brazil.

Siebold's ambition to explore unknown worlds, his wide outlook and his interest in natural history must have appealed to the Governor-General, who himself had a lively interest in natural sciences. Van der Capellen considered the young Siebold as "our second Kaempfer and Thunberg". He gave the mission to Japan – in Siebold's own words – a "grossnifitige", or magnanimous support, first financially, enabling Siebold to buy the necessary instruments, materials and books, and later, in a unique gesture, by providing a small staff. Two assistants were appointed: the pharmacist Heinrich Bürger for chemical, mineralogical and geological surveys and Lieutenant Carl Hubert de Villeneuve who would draw the different objects collected by Siebold.

We may conclude that Siebold was scientifically well trained, had personal ambition and the support of the Governor-General. This was however not sufficient to make the mission successful. Equally important was support in Japan. When Siebold arrived in Nagasaki in August 1823, he had in this respect a fortunate starting position compared with most of his predecessors. Captains such as Doeff and Cock Blomhoff had established, during their long stays at Dejima earlier that century, a relatively free accessibility to European medical knowledge. Even though the Dutch could only leave Dejima under very restricted conditions it had become a custom to consult the Dejima doctor in severe cases of illness in Nagasaki. A limited number of Japanese physicians had received permission to visit Dejima regularly. Siebold could in fact build on the network created earlier that century by the Dejima captains and "doctors."

The whole enterprise therefore depended largely on the confidence that Siebold could create as a physician. In that sense he turned out to be competent too. His fame spread soon to Edo where the main centre of "Hollandologists" was located. From the correspondence of one of them, Takano Chôei, it is evident that they realized that a prominent doctor now practiced at Dejima, a doctor, who even had official permission to visit patients outside Dejima! Many *Rangakusha* looked forward to a trip to Nagasaki, since, according to Takano, "one year study in Edo is only a fight on tatami. But even half a year in Nagasaki is fighting with real weapons."

This brings us to what seems to me an essential part of the success of Siebold's mission in Japan: the foundation of a school. Siebold informed his German patron Nees von Esenbeck just 3 months after his arrival that he regularly gave lessons in medicine and natural history to a group of first-rate Japanese students and interpreters, In a publication of 1824 he referred to that school as the Collegium Medicum. It was frequented by promising pupils such as Chôan Minato, Kôsai Yoshio, Junzô Mima, Kaisô Hirai and Ryôsai Kô .

It was not easy to start the school under the restrictions imposed on contacts between the Japanese and the Dutch. Siebold wanted to teach medicine to students in town, particularly in relation to his practical lessons. The Nagasaki governor complied-with the request only after the intercession of the interpreter Narabayashi Sôken. From then on Siebold, accompanied by seven interpreters, went three times a week to the private schools of Narabayashi and Yoshiô, where he taught the students and demonstrated and treated patients.

As the number of students increased, the governor gave permission for the school to move to an area near Nagasald, in the valley of Narutaki. This school, known as *Narutaki Juku*, was the first *shijuku or* private school established by a European during the Tokugawa period. As in other *shijuku*, there was no fixed curriculum in Siebold's school, but one can expect that with someone like Siebold the teaching was systematic. In the beginning he taught mainly the theory and practice of medicine and natural history. Pharmacology was added to the program in the

Narutaki school. Siebold did not teach just by reading; he also introduced demonstrations of medical and surgical treatment.

In connection with his own scientific interests Siebold adopted an exceptional teaching method. It covered a larger area than western medicine and sciences since the students were assigned papers on a variety of other subjects, to be written in Dutch. Students received a certificate on leaving the school, on condition that they would write a *dissertatio inauguralis* – as Siebold called it – after returning home. They would then present it to him during the journey to Edo. The subject was given by Siebold and often covered little-known ethnological subjects such as "The oldest history and mythology of Japan," "Lists of temples and churches at Edo and Miyako," "Description of Japanese chronology," or "Ethics for Japanese women." Sometimes the topics concerned only a translation or summary of a Japanese text. Even at his departure Siebold gave instructions to his students to send him theses on certain subjects. About 40 theses are known, 11 of which were included in Siebold's main work *Nippon*. In this context one should realize that students at Narutaki Juku were usually older than those in most of the other private schools and that they were not preparing for a career. Siebold's students were usually already well educated and experienced physicians.

The gathering of information reached a height during the court journey from February to June 1826. Siebold was able to choose the participants in the journey as he wished. Bilrger was chosen as secretary instead of one the higher-ranking Dejima employees who usually accompanied the captain. Unfortunately Siebold was not able to include de Villeneuve, but his task was taken over by the capable painter Keiga Kawahara. Siebold had won over the leader of the journey, Genshô Kawasaki, to his scientific enterprise. This probably resulted in the relatively large number of personal Japanese assistants who could accompany Siebold: first of all the diligent student Ryôsai Kô, then his servants Benoske and Komaki (charged with drying plants and preparing animal skins), and finally a gardener. The students Minomiya Keisakôu and Ishii Sôken, who had not received permission to go, were included in the retinue as servants of the interpreters. Siebold's 'research staff' and Kawasaki's willingness made it possible to make many personal observations on natural history and geology during the trip and to go outside the prescribed route.

During the journey Siebold experienced what he called 'unusual favors' from Japanese scholars. For instance in Nagoya he met the botanists Hôbun Mizutani (with whom Siebold had already corresponded) and Itô Keisuke. These men searched for rare plants, dried them and drew them for Siebold's collection. On his return to Dejima Siebold persuaded Itô to come to Nagasaki. Itô helped Siebold to identify about 2000 plants. In Edo Siebold met another person with whom he had already corresponded, namely the court physician Ishisaka Setsu. The latter's treatise on acupuncture and moxa was published by Siebold in 1833 in the proceedings of the Batavian Society for Arts and Sciences. He also met in Edo the geographers Monagi Tokunai, who told him about the unknown northern parts of Japan, and Takahashi Sakuzaemon, who presented him with a secret map of Japan.

Siebold never asked for money for his consultations and advice. He exchanged his knowledge and experience for material objects, as for instance he did in Edo with the ophthalmologist Habu Genseki. Siebold revealed the secrets of the drug belladonna to Genseki in exchange for a *kosode,* a state dress with the crest of the Tokugawa family. The possession of forbidden goods, such as this state dress and the map of Japan, and his correspondence with Takahashi, provoked the so-called Siebold affair, resulting in his expulsion from Japan at the end of December 1829.

After his return to the Netherlands in July 1830 Siebold settled in Leiden to begin the second part of his scientific enterprise, the publication of the results of his activities in Japan. Siebold's publications during his stay on Dejima were limited, but they had already attracted the attention of European scholars. The scientific community would now really hear from him as he concentrated on his magnum opus, the trilogy *Nippon, Flora Japonica* and *Fauna Japonica.* For his researches Siebold wanted to be in the vicinity of 'his' collections. The natural history part had been collected by order of the government and as state property was housed in the National Herbarium and the National Natural History Museum, both in Leiden. In 1837 the government bought Siebold's ethnological collection, which was then, with other Dutch collections from Japan, also housed in Leiden. For that reason he settled in this university town (although he disliked the Dutch climate), and chose not a professorial career but a purely scientific one, without the burden of teaching. Choosing teaching, as he wrote to his mother in 1830, would be like "moving from a horse to a donkey".

Siebold's arrival in the Netherlands occurred during a period when the national treasury suffered from the heavy expenses caused by the Belgian revolt. And although Siebold had excellent protection at the royal court, the government was not able to finance the gigantic operation that Siebold had in mind. The actual purchase of Siebold's collection in 1837 came 6 years after the government agreed to Siebold's proposal. It was not only the ambitious format of the publications and the many colored figures and maps included in them that made the costs so high, but also the creation of a personal staff. The project included, apart from a number of artists and lithographers, in particular Ko-Tsing-Tsang and Johann Joseph Hoffmann. The Chinese co-worker accompanied Siebold from Java and assisted in his philological studies. The Würzburger Hoffmann, an opera singer with philological training, assisted in the translation of Japanese sources. He established another Leiden-Würzburg relationship when he was appointed as the first professor of Japanese at Leiden university in 1855 (Fig. 1).

Since governmental support was not sufficient, Siebold developed another aspect of research management, namely fundraising. In order to raise interest in his work and to find subscribers for his publications he made a tour in 1834/5 to Saint Petersburg, Moscow, Berlin, Dresden, Prague, Vienna and Munich. Stimulated by the support he experienced Siebold returned to Leiden and continued his activities. In the meantime the first issues of his work had appeared: *Nippon* and *Fauna Japonica* in 1833 and *Flora Japonica* in 1834.

The *Fauna* and *Flora Japonica* once more demonstrate Siebold's ability to plan and coordinate a large project and to obtain the cooperation of top-ranking scientists. For his botanical work he could count upon the support of his old German patrons Dö11inger and Nees von Esenbeck. In the final publication of the first volumes of the *Flora Japonica* he cooperated with Joseph Gerhard Zuccarini, professor of botany at Munich. An important initiative related to his botanical research was the foundation of a society to import plants from Japan. This private enterprise was a joint venture with the Leiden botany professor, Karl Blume, director of the National Herbarium, whom Siebold had met earlier in Batavia as director of the botanical garden Buitenzorg.

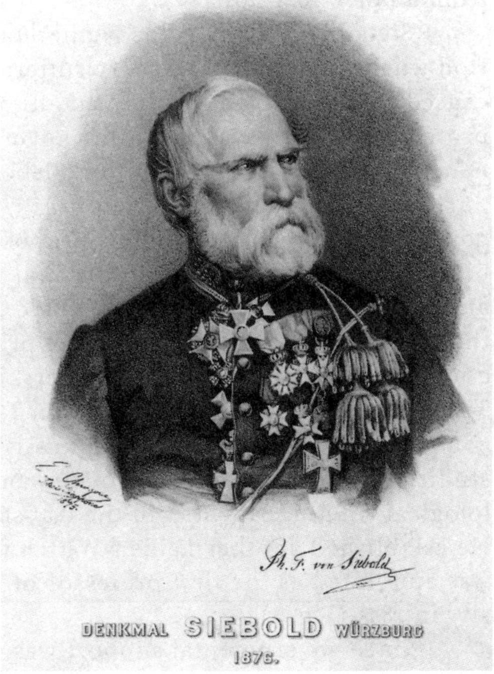

Fig. 1. Philip Franz von Siebold

For publication of the zoological material Siebold depended heavily on cooperation with the directors of the National Natural History Museum in Leiden, C.J. Temminck and H. Schlegel, and their custodian W. de Haan. Since Siebold was not well versed in zoology he was less involved in this publication but generously put his material and notes at the disposal of these men. In this respect we must praise Siebold. Whenever scholars were interested in aspects of his work they found a ready ear, as the Leiden anatomist Gerard Sandifort experienced when he was able to complete his physical anthropological studies with the (first) description of Japanese skulls from Siebold's collection.

I have restricted my survey to Siebold's first visit to Japan and his work in Leiden, because these periods show him in his full glory as a scholar and, as I hope to have convinced you, as a full-blown modern research manager. In that sense he is still a shining example for future cooperation on his career stretching from Würzburg to Nagasaki to Leiden.

CHAPTER 11

German Medicine in Japan*

G. Keil

In attempting to show the influence of German medicine on Japan it is best to start from a morphological and structurally orientated point of view. The latter has been reflected in illustrated works and has been influenced by China since the Tang dynasty. Japan was culturally dominated by China from the first century after the birth of Christ. The beginning of the influence of German thinking in the natural sciences is shown best in morphological knowledge transferred by pictures. In modern times, a different perception of morphological knowledge can be seen in China and Japan: beginning in the early eighteenth century, everything began to change in Japanese medicine.

During the Tang dynasty Chinese, which belongs to the Tibet-Tai language group, had developed into a monosyllabic root isolating language to such a degree that problems of comprehension arose. These difficulties could be eliminated neither with the help of intonation (principle of tonality) nor by grammatical or semantic rules for the position of words within a sentence. The mono-, di- and triphthongal monosyllabic words developed many homophones, particularly because of a common nasal ending. These homophones were all pronounced the same way and had the same intonation. Therefore, phonetic notation was no help. For this reason, the pictorial writing practiced in the early Shang dynasty was maintained. Ideograms with the Shang dynasty type of spelling could be formed with brushes and further developed by synthesis. Inverted signs, borrowed signs and symbolic combinations to which phonetic or semantic functions had been assigned appeared next to simple and symbolic pictures. (The same development occurred in colloquial speech through the addition

* Lecture given on the occasion of the meeting of the German Society of Legal Medicine in Würzburg on May 29, 1997.

of supplementary signs: the so-called *Lauter* and *Deuter*.) The ambiguity of terms that resulted from this development could hardly be abolished by composing elements with several lexemes and symbols.

This very complex system, consisting of synonymous compositions, *Lauter/Deuter* combinations, an intonation of four to seven stresses and no specific word-order, functioned because of the commitment to tradition. It helped to keep the system stable for more than 1000 years and was also very consistent. The way of thinking was influenced by deeply rooted, speculative symbols and it followed pictographic–symbolic associations. These were not only installed within historic and symbolic combinations but were also based on symbols existing within semantic fields.

In medicine one can also find a common tradition of images based on speculation. Their stability, going back to the traditions of the Tang dynasty, were generally accepted in the medical sector, and interpretations (with little or no reference to reality) had their origin in symbolic-fictional image patterns. Medical discussions dealt with questions like the following: why does the spleen – situated on the right side – resemble the sole of a shoe? Why is the structure of the liver – situated on the left side – similar to the structure of a leaf? People were also preoccupied (of course in a speculative and symbolic way) with the problem of the three heating cords that started from the heart. Finally, Chinese scientists regarded the kidney on the right as a store – similar to a testicle – for sperm. They did not agree that there was an organ which filters water and discharges urine to the bladder.

In Japan, scientists thought in the same way as their Chinese colleagues. Similarity in the specialist literature and education was one reason for similar thinking about the meanings of symbolic images and is also why emblematic patterns were associated too. It has to be noted that the pictograms of Chinese notation, supported by images, form an identical and ideographic pattern of reference. An identical metaphoric system based on symbols and an interpretation helped by images appeared in the speculative theories of China and Japan.

The adoption of German medicine in Japan coincided with Germany's first important colonial period. In 1602 some areas of Indonesia became part of the *Heiliges Römisches Reich deutscher Nation*, in 1624 Taiwan was annexed, in 1612 Nieuw Amsterdam (which is now New York) was founded, and in 1641 the artificial island of Dejima in the bay of Nagasaki was taken. The quick spread of Catholicism in Japan which began in 1543 ended in a massacre of Christians and was the reason for Japan's isolation from 1640 onward. The representatives of the German Empire were allowed to install a trading post on Dejima and to run a business establishment in Nagasaki harbour. After the 30 Years' War had ended and the peace treaty of Osnabrück had been signed, the Dutch ran the German colonies and Nagasaki thus came under Dutch administration. The Japanese interpreter, who (apart from some seasonal exceptions) was the only person in touch with the German-Dutch foreigners, called himself *Rangaku* or *Rangakusha* (Dutch–scholar). For the first time, the strict isolation of Japan was overcome by western, in particular German, medicine with the help of this *Rangaku*.

The adoption of European and in particular German medicine in Japan started in about 1660. The whole transfer of knowledge can be divided into four phases.

Procedures using illustrations were adopted first. Occidental diagrams used for demonstration purposes followed the pathological *Dreibilderserie* (series of three pictures, influenced by the Würzburg School) or the anatomical *Fünfbilderserie* (series of five pictures). These drawings and their message relating to the late Middle Ages slipped Zo shi into the "remarks on the viscera". The diagrams succeeded as an independent structural system in the Würzburg-Prague model by providing a woodcut whose iconographic message was completed by comments. The whole procedure not only corresponded extremely well with the Prague model but also matched Ortolf's "Wundenmann" of Würzburg. Some famous examples may be mentioned.

The "corpse of a decapitated criminal" ("Leiche eines enthaupteten Verbrechers") was demonstrated by Yamawaki Toyo, physician-in-ordinary to the Emperor of Kyoto. This medical doctor published his findings in 1754 in writing and in block printing. The same was done by Tomon, a court physician who dissected a female criminal according to the German pattern. Afterwards, Tomon noted his dissection findings on a *Makimono*, a transverse parchment paper. Brain, eyes, chest, abdomen and skeleton were sketched. Although the notes go beyond traditional Chinese knowledge, they seem to be imperfect or "very primitive", from our point of view.

The second stage in the transfer of German medical knowledge to Japan consisted not merely of imitation but of illustrative work with supplementary diagrams and with translated texts.

The first European specialist literature translated into Japanese was Johann Remmelin's *Catoptrum microcosmicum*. This work, which first appeared in Augsburg in 1613, follows Vesalius's *Fabrica*. Remmelin dissected the body into different layers. Copperplate prints based on drawings by Remmelin were prepared by Lukas Kilian. The (German or rather) Dutch edition was published in 1634 under the title *Ontleding des menschelijke lichaems*. The latter version interested the Japanese population living on Dejima, who translated the book into Japanese. Motoki Ryoi, who was born in Nagasaki and died in Tokyo in 1697, was the translator, and Takei Rippo made the woodcuts. *Catoptrum microcosmicum* circulated in this way and in handwritten form for more than 100 years. A reprint produced in Tokyo was put on the market in 1772, edited by Suzuki Soun and Shimizu Go.

The third phase of German–Japanese knowledge transfer is characterized by the compilation of texts based on German texts. Instead of merely taking the original books or imitating the illustrations in them, the texts were revised, independently illustrated, and summed up in compendiums.

As an example, I would like to refer to Johann Adam Kulms from Breslau, whose anatomic charts (*Anatomischen Tabellen*) were published in Danzig in 1722. The Dutch translation by Gerhard Dicten was finished in 1734, while the Japanese revision entitled *Kaitai Shinsho* appeared in Tokyo in 1773. The Japanese version of Adam Kulms *Anatomic Chart* edited by Gempaku Sugita and Junan Nakagawa was part of a collection of another eight original German books. Genjo illustrated all three volumes in one book of plates made from woodcuts.

The fourth and last stage of Japan's adoption of German medicine was achieved through Otsuku Gentaku, a student of Gempaku Sugita. In 1798, 130 years after the exchange of knowledge had begun, he introduced his *Chotei Katai Shinsho* text. In addition to an atlas volume this monumental work consisted of 13 volumes of text.

Beginning in the seventeenth century and ending in the eighteenth century Japanese medicine became German or, in other words, it became very modern and occidental. The distance from traditional Chinese medicine, which was still using its symbolic language and speculative symbols, was striking. In the eighteenth century, Japanese medicine was based on the image. This can be proved by looking at some oft-repeated phrases. In the eighteenth century medicine in Japan offered "Dutch images" and began to draw and arrange illustrations. However, Japanese medicine used the leading imaging procedures of the time and did not copy the traditional image patterns, but rather documented experimental findings with the help of the most modern media. "He drew what he had seen" is how Japanese medicine referred to the involved artist.

Chinese medicine still persisted in its traditional limits and fought fiercely against the exchange of knowledge until 1800 or even later. It used the argument that in western medicine the liver was considered to be situated on the right side while in China, as everybody knew, the liver was on the left, Chinese medicine consequently defended and refined its traditional links; it also referred to special truths and postulated incontestable special findings. On the other hand, Japanese medicine, which had been completely isolated, moved westwards and adopted international standards. It strove for the truth. Its motto was: "The truth is the same everywhere".

To describe the aggressive process of the detachment of Japanese medicine from Chinese medicine I would like to quote from the monumental *Chotei Katai Shinsho*, where Gentaku Otsuki states: "What is described in classical Chinese medicine is great and wonderful but it has no truth at all." He adds that probably only a tenth is true and that this small part is presented in a confused form. The statements simply couldn't be understood and therefore Gentaku Otsuki concluded that there was nothing else to be done than to banish Chinese medicine.

"*Doitsu bongaku*": Through Dutch intervention Japanese medicine became German and thus international in the eighteenth century. While the country known as the land of the rising sun remained in self-chosen political and cultural isolation, its medicine developed towards international, particularly German, standards.

Japanese medicine in the eighteenth century respected the Germans and the Dutch highly. Again, I would like to refer to Gentaku Otsuki, as a contemporary of this time, by quoting the following from his book: "Dutch images (are) extremely exact ... correspond to facts and one may check their statements by means of experiments. The findings are totally identical with Dutch images". Further enthusiastic praise is given to the Germans, and this might be considered to represent the views of Japanese medical doctors from the seventeenth to the twentieth century.

The Germans! The Dutch! "What these people realized with their intellect, their heart and their hands is so miraculous that one can compare it to a prodigy of nature."

In the eighteenth century, it was assumed that the German influence that started from Dejima – and in particular from Nagasaki – continued. The first person who should be mentioned is the medical doctor Engelbert Kämpfer, who was in the service of the government of the Dutch East Indies from 1690 to 1692 and who lived on Dejima. He was famous for his interest in the natural sciences. His book *History and Description of Japan* (1712) was published posthumously in 1727 (and in 1777/79) and became the essential book of the century for knowledge about Japan. This work in two volumes influenced politics when Japan stepped out of its isolation in 1854–1861, and it kept its international standing up to that time.

Philipp Franz von Siebold, from the eastern Franconia – lower Rhine area, was employed as a a medical doctor by the Bavarians but started to work for the Dutch in 1820. He was educated by students of his grandfather in Würzburg and after changing his employer he served on Dejima from 1823–1829. Japan owes to him vaccination, couching and the installation of pharmacies according to the most modern rules of pharmacy. Like Kaempfer, Siebold stressed botany; his geographical maps covered the Japanese islands, and his collections of artwork and natural specimens are well regarded. Parts of these collections can be seen now in the Würzburger Siebold Museum. Siebold's "Nippon-Archive" is extensive, although it consists of only seven parts. It describes Japan and its protectorates.

The main influence on Japanese medicine has to be assigned to the German medical doctor Erwin von Baelz. He was no longer employed by the Dutch but worked for the Emperor. He worked not in Dejima-Nagasaki but in Edo (now Tokyo) where the Emperor lived. This Prussian medical officer took over the old medical school near Edo. When he was making changes at the school, the Charité in Berlin served as an example for him. In 1878 this medical school resembling the Berlin Charité became part of the recently founded University of Tokyo. It was characteristic of Baelz's students and their descendants (among them the famous Hakura Hashimoto) that they went to Germany for their postgraduate studies, especially if they were interested in undertaking research work. They also came to Germany to perfect their clinical work.

Engelbert Kämpfer, Philipp Franz von Siebold, Erwin Baelz and many other medical doctors stole the limelight from the hundreds of people dealing with texts in the seventeenth and eighteenth centuries. These people translated medical texts, and their great work should not be overlooked.

I would like to end by quoting an anonymous spokesman for a group of collaborators who started translating German books as early as 1700 or thereabouts.

> We [that is the writer and another ten colleagues] have been busy for some years with the translation of a German book ... German language sounds strange and the symbols bend over like nails... they look like legs of a mosquito ... and they never mean the same ... it is hard to understand the grammar ...Germany is famous in the world and particularly its medicine ... Its books of therapy dominate the whole world because they are splendid. But they are hard to understand. ... The members of my family have been medical doctors for generations ... I was educated to become a doctor when I was a child ... I studied the German book together with some colleges patiently and permanently. We helped each other and we discussed ... We dissected according to the dissection method explained in the book ... the text seemed to be consequent ... gradually the contents of each chapter becomes clearer.

Suggested Reading

1. Auer E, Schnell B (1993) Der "Wundenmann". Ein traumatologisches Schema in der Tradition der "Wundarznei" des Ortolf von Baierland. In: Keil G, Mayer JG, Naser C (eds) Ein teutsch puech machen. Untersuchungen zur landessprachlichen Vermittlung medizinischen Wissens. Ludwig Reichert, Wiesbaden, pp 349-401 (Ortolf-Studien I; Wissensliteratur im Mittelalter. Schriften des Sonderforschungsbereichs 226 Würzburg/Eichstätt, 11)

2. Bälz T (1930) Das Leben eines deutschen Arztes im erwachenden Japan: Tagebücher, Briefe, Berichte. In: Bälz E (ed). Spemann, Stuttgart
3. Ebert J, Beireis U (eds) (1995) Auf den Spuren Siebolds in Würzburg und Japan. Siebold-Gesellschaft, Würzburg, pp 38-47 (Katalog zur Eröffnungsausstellung des Siebold-Museums, Würzburg 3.7.–2.10.1995)
4. Keil G (1986) Dreibilderserie, in: Lexikon des Mittelalters, vol. III, Artemis, München, p 1373ff
5. Keil G (1990) Ortolf's chirurgischer Traktat und das Aufkommen der medizinischen Demonstrationszeichnung. In: Harms W (ed) Text und Bild, Bild und Text. DFG-Symposion 1988. Metzler, Stuttgart, pp 117, 120ff, 134, 137–149, 216–221, 347ff, Figs. 41-52 (Germanistische Symposien, Berichtsband 11)
6. Holler M (1977) Vorlesung zur Medizin- und Wissenschaftsgeschichte Ostasiens. University of Würzburg, Wintersemester 1977/1978, No. 613
7. van der Pas PW (1973) Engelbert Kaempfer. In: Gillispie CC (ed) Dictionary of scientific biography. vol VII. Scribner's Sons, New York, pp 204b–206a
8. Schottlaender F (1928) Erwin von Baelz 1849–1913. Leben und Wirken eines deutschen Arztes in Japan. Ausland und Heimat Verlag, Stuttgart (Schriften des Deutschen Auslands-Instituts Stuttgart, Reihe D: Biographica und Denkwürdigkeiten, vol 1)
9. Scurla H (ed) (1968) Reisen in Nippon. Berichte deutscher Forscher des 18. und 19. Jahrhunderts aus Japan: Engelbert Kaempfer, Georg Heinrich von Langsdorff, Philipp Franz von Siebold. Verlag Nation, Berlin
10. Seidel G (1995) Studien zur Geschichte der Hashimoto-Thyroiditis. Medical Thesis, University of Würzburg
11. Wagenseil F (1959) Die drei ersten unter europäischem ([deutschem bzw.] holländischem) Einfluß entstandenen japanischen Anatomiebücher. Sudhoffs Arch 43:61–85 (with the support of the DFG and in collaboration with Teizo Ogawa, Tokyo)

CHAPTER 12

German Physicians in Japan: Personal, Medical and Cultural Characteristics

E. Kraas

For Japan, 1868 saw the beginning of a new age which came to be known as the Meiji Restoration Period. The 16-year-old Tenno had taken over the government, moved his residence from Kyoto to Tokyo, and introduced reforms in all walks of life, in accordance with the maxim "knowledge from the whole world must be acquired". This was to include western medicine. With regard to the physicians who were to be appointed, the recommendations of the foreign policy adviser, Guido Fridolin Verbeck (1830–1898) (Fig. 1), were followed. He proposed German physicians, because, as was required, they did not come from a republican state. On 11 July 1870 the Prussian Premier, Max von Brandt (1835–1920), was thus able to draw up a 3-year contract for two physicians. He recommended to the Prussian government two senior army medical officers who, due to the outbreak of the Franco-Prussian War a few days later, were unable to start their journey until May 1871. They reached Yokohama on 25 August 1871 via New York, Salt Lake City and San Francisco.

Who were these Prussian doctors? Major Leopold Müller (1822–1893) (Fig. 2) of the medical corps was a lecturer at the Friedrich-Wilhelm Academy of Surgeons and from 1857–1867 Inspector General of the army and military hospitals in Haiti. The internist was naval medical officer Theodor Eduard Hoffmann (1837–1894), whom Müller had come to know and highly regard while at the Berlin Medical Academy.

Müller and Hoffmann had to teach Japanese students the entire medical curriculum through an interpreter and without any textbooks. They were confronted with 300 students who expected their new teachers to add extensively to the knowledge of Chinese medicine they had already acquired. Müller examined them and discovered that none of them possessed sufficient knowledge of anatomy and physiology. They were therefore all re-

Fig. 1. Guido Fidolin Verbeck (1830–1898)

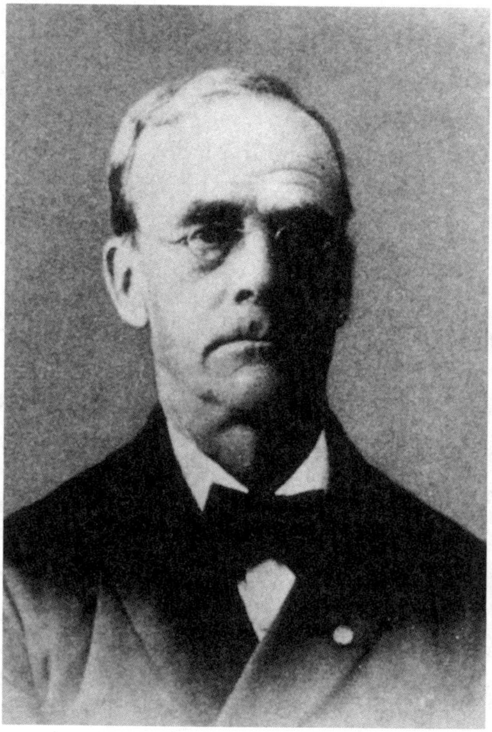

quired to repeat the first semester. After 4 months, 59 of them were left, and only 29 took the examination. The study course took 8 years. The first 3 years consisted of so-called preparatory courses, which were followed by ten semesters at the Academy. From 1873 on it was possible to give the courses in German. Latin was a compulsory subject. The Tokyo Medical School was renamed Kaiserliche Medizinische Akademie (Imperial Medical Academy). A third teacher was engaged, Karl Friedrich Dönitz (1838–1912), whose teaching covered the whole field of anatomy, including lectures on cadavers which constituted the beginning of forensic medicine. In 1873 Max von Brandt and Leopold Müller founded the German East Asian Society for Natural History and Ethnology.

At the request of the Japanese government, Müller and Hoffmann extended their contracts for a further year. On their departure they were highly honored and presented with generous gifts. They had founded a university along German lines and cre-

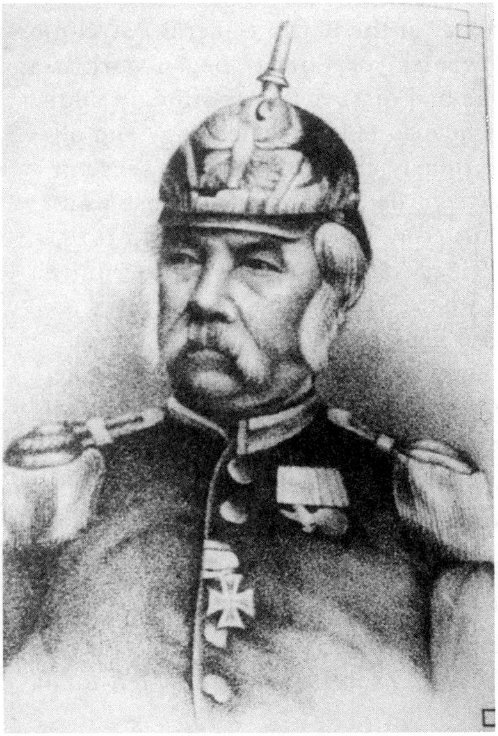

Fig. 2. Leopold Müller (1822–1893)

ated the basis for lasting Japanese–German relations. Hoffmann wrote the first study on beriberi, which of course reflected the knowledge of the day. Ten years after his return from Japan, Müller published an article in the *Deutsche Rundschau* on his impressions and his experience there.

The successor to Müller and Hoffmann in Tokyo was the surgeon Emil August Wilhelm Schultze (1840–1924), who was the senior assistant doctor in the surgical department at the Charité Hospital in Berlin. On a study trip to England he had become acquainted with Lister's antiseptic treatment of wounds. The first ovariectomy, which he carried out in 1881, is still remembered today. His students regarded Schultze as "polite, hard-working and eager for knowledge". He renewed his contract for a further 3 years. During his period in office he became Dean of the Medical Academy, which was renamed the Imperial University (Kaiserliche Universität) in 1877. The first examinations were also carried out during this period.

In 1875 the senior lecturer at the Berlin General Polyclinic, Albrecht Ludwig Agathon Wernich (1843–1892), began work as an internist in Tokyo. In 1874 he had discovered ergotine. In addition to his own special field he also taught Gynecology and obstetrics. He worked conscientiously and with a strong sense of duty but remained reserved towards the Japanese, whose ways were foreign to him. He returned to Germany in 1878. In 1876, Hans Paul Gerhard Giercke (1847–1886) took over from Dönitz and spent 3 years in Tokyo, where he gave the first lectures on comparative anatomy. Johann Ernst Tiegel (1849–1889), appointed Professor of Physiology in 1877, also taught pathology, hygiene and forensic medicine. His most important student was Kenji Osawa (1852–1927), now considered to be "the father of Japanese physiology". Tiegel had studied under Hermann von Helmholtz and Emil Du Bois Reymond. He stayed in Tokyo until 1883.

In 1876, the internist Erwin Otto Eduard Baelz (1849–1913) (Fig. 3) was sent to Tokyo by the Japanese envoy in Berlin. He had been assistant doctor under Professor Wunderlich (1815–1877) in Leipzig and became professor before he left for Ja-

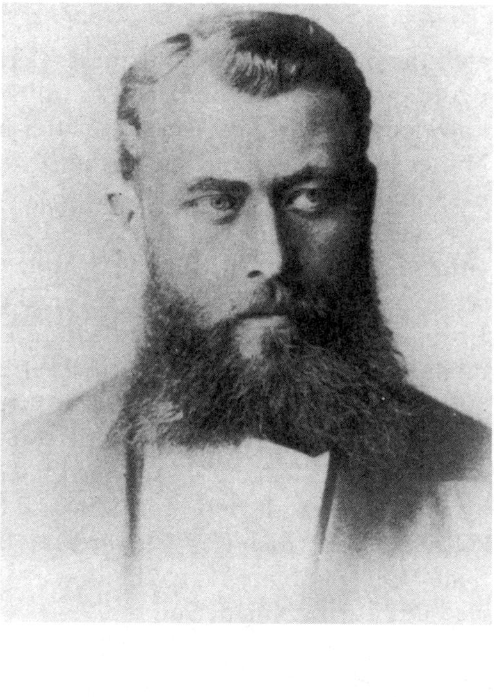

Fig. 3. Erwin Otto Eduard Bälz (1849–1913)

pan. This appointment meant to him, as he put it, "the fulfillment of one of his most cherished dreams". In addition to internal medicine he also taught Gynecology and obstetrics. Later he was the first to teach psychiatry. In 1880, his contract was renewed for another 4 years, and then again until 1902. In 1888, he married a Japanese woman. Besides teaching and practicing medicine, he was also interested in infectious diseases in Japan, the prevention of epidemics and the effectiveness of thermal baths, based on his own experience in Kusatsu. Anthropological studies, conducted with his assistant Miura, led to the discovery of blue spot. His reputation brought him patients from as far away as China and India. Since 1890 Baelz had been private physician to the Emperor's family. He gave his farewell lecture in 1902, but stayed on in Japan until 1905. His students hailed him as the father of Japanese medicine. In 1907, a bronze statue of him was erected in the university grounds. After his return home, he was awarded the Commander's Cross of the Order of the Crown, which was associated with the life peerage. On the 20th anniversary of his death, the town of Kusatsu set up a commemorative stone and on the 150th anniversary of his death his birthplace, Bietigheim, was given a copy of this memorial. There are strong cultural links between the two towns.

The last German surgeon to go to Tokyo, Julius Scriba (1848–1905), arrived in 1881. After 1 year working under Langenbeck in Berlin, he joined Gustav Simon in Freiburg and took his final examinations, entitling him to become a professor, there in 1879. In Tokyo he lectured not only on surgery but also on dermatology, ophthalmology and forensic medicine. He was regarded as the best surgeon in the whole of Japan, carrying out the first nephrectomy there in 1888. Patients were referred to him from all East Asian capitals. He had a Japanese wife and three children. In 1893, the Grand Duke of Hesse awarded him the title of professor. In the same year he became physician to the Imperial German Mission. In 1901 he left the University, and in 1902 was appointed head surgeon in a Tokyo hospital. Scriba also carried out anthropological studies. The Technical University in Darmstadt owns a collection of Japanese mosses and woody plants to his early love of botany. When he died in 1905, his wife and children stayed on in Japan.

Josef Hugo Vincenz Disse (1852–1912), the last German anatomist to work in Tokyo, taught histology, embryology and topographic and pathological anatomy. After 7 years' work, there he returned to Germany.

From 1872 onwards, German physicians also lectured at other medical schools. From 1872 to 1876, Ferdinand Adalbert Junker von Langegg (1828–1901), who, in addition to his own subject, surgery, also taught anatomy, obstetrics, pathology and later internal medicine and therapy, was a lecturer at the newly founded medical school in Kyoto. He invented an apparatus for anesthesia. His translations of Japanese literature and essays on Japanese painting show where his interests lay. The Austrian, Albrecht von

Roretz (1846–1884), lectured in all fields of medicine from 1877 until 1880 in Nagoya, then for 1 year in Kanazawa and subsequently for a further 3 years in Yamagata.

From 1877 to 1881, Heinrich Botho Scheube (1853–1923) lectured in Kyoto; in addition to his special subject, internal medicine, he also taught physiology, histology and diagnostics. In addition to several studies on beriberi, Scheube also wrote on other medical subjects. He was particularly interested in the indigenous population, the Ainos. His extensive ethnological collection can be found in the Ethnology Museum in Leipzig.

Richard Wunsch (1869–1911) was the last German physician of this generation. He did not work as a university lecturer, however, but was Imperial Physician to the Emperor in Seoul. On Baelz's advice, he then went to Tokyo as mission physician from 1905 to 1908. He was not able to fulfill his intention to set up a practice there as, from 1908 onwards, foreign doctors were only allowed to practice if they had Japanese qualifications. For this reason he went to work as a senior hospital physician in Tsingtau, where he died in 1911.

To sum up, it can be said that all the medical scholars who were sent to Japan had both special qualifications and general medical knowledge beyond their own fields. Moreover, all of them had diverse interests outside medicine. Above all, they took a great interest in the problems of the host country, which led to close ties with their students.

Let us now look at the Japanese side. Once the decision to appoint German lecturers had been made, the first Japanese students were sent to study in Germany. One of these was Kensai Ikeda. After his return in 1876, he became director of the Polyclinic under Schultze. It was the aim of the Japanese government to replace the Germans with Japanese lecturers. The best were

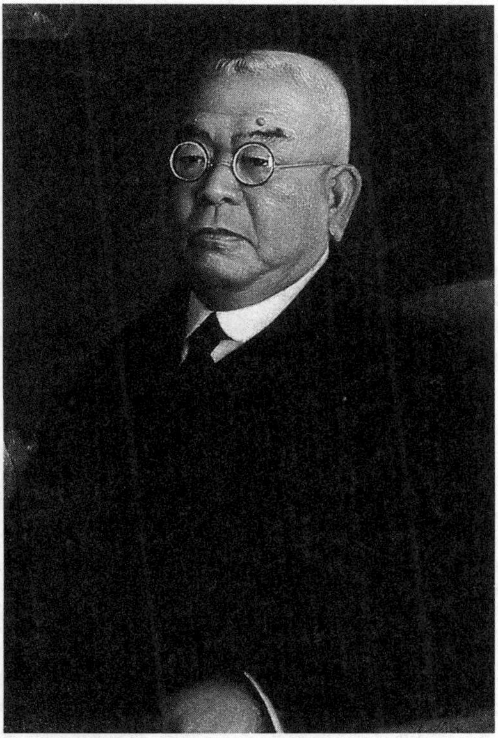

Fig. 4. Shibasaburo Kitasato (1856–1931)

therefore sent to Germany after completion of their studies for further specialized training. This process began in 1885 with the arrival in Berlin of Shibasaburo Kitasato (1856–1931) (Fig. 4). For 5 years he studied the field of epidemic control under Robert Koch (1843–1910) (Fig. 5). Working for Koch, Kitasato experienced his first success with the production of a pure culture of anthrax bacilli. His stay was extended and he worked with Behring (1847–1917) on tetanus vaccination. In 1892, he went back to Japan and founded a private laboratory with German equipment. His scientific reports were published in German medical journals. He kept in touch with Robert Koch, and their professional relationship reached its peak in 1908, when Kitasato gave Koch a very honorable welcome in Tokyo.

Sahachiro Hata (1873–1938), who had been trained by Kitasato since 1898, became Paul Ehrlich's co-worker (1854–1915) (Fig. 6). In 1910, Hata's investigations led to the development of a new medical product against syphilis, sold under the brand name

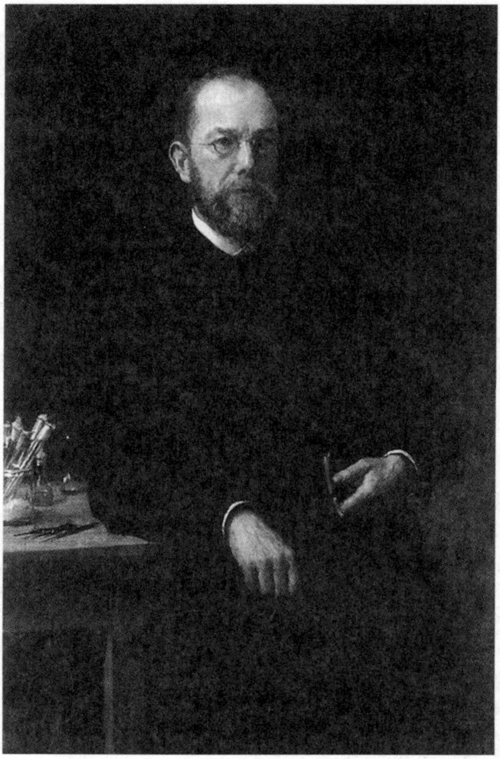

Fig. 5. Robert Koch (1843–1931)

Salvarsan. Moriharu Miura (1857–1916) worked for several years with the world-famous pathologist Virchow (1821–1902) in his Berlin institute. Back in Japan, he became the first director of the Institute for Pathological Anatomy. The Japanese continued to come to Germany, preferably to Berlin and Freiburg. As reminders of successful teamwork the terms Aschoff-Tawara knots and Masugi nephritis are still known today.

Rintaro Mori (1863–1922), better known as Ogai Mori (Fig. 7), was one of the first generation of Japanese physicians to study in Germany. In 1877 he began his medical training, became an army medical officer and was posted to Germany to study hygiene and military sanitation. From 1884 to 1888, he spent 1 year each in Leipzig, Dresden, Munich and Berlin. He was the first Japanese to serve as an army medical officer in Berlin. In addition to the study of his special subject, he was fascinated by European literature. In his career in his home country, he reached the most senior position as the director of the medical department of

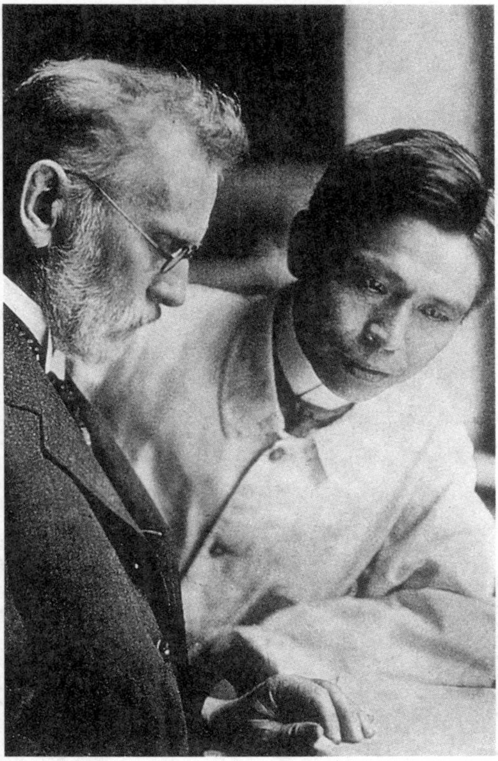

Fig. 6. Sahachiro Hata (1873–1938) and Paul Ehrlich (1854–1915)

the War Office. He founded a journal on hygiene and another on medicine. His literary career began at the same time. He wrote short novels and translated European literature. In 1908, on the occasion of Robert Koch's visit, he wrote two one-act plays. Between 1911 and 1913, he translated both parts of Goethe's *Faust*.

As already mentioned, in the early years gynecology and obstetrics were taught by German surgeons and internists. In 1880 the development of gynecology as a separate subject was slowly beginning. Ikujiro Sakurai founded a school of midwifery and taught European medicine there. In the same year, I. Shimizu came to Germany, followed by Masakiyo Ogata (1864–1919), who took his doctorate in Freiburg and then worked with Hegel in Berlin. Mizu Takahashi, a female student of Sakurai's, came to Berlin in 1890 for further training. Yoichi Ikeda (born in 1858) was in Germany around 1900. He later referred to himself as "one of the oldest gynecologists to have the pleasure of studying with German lecturers".

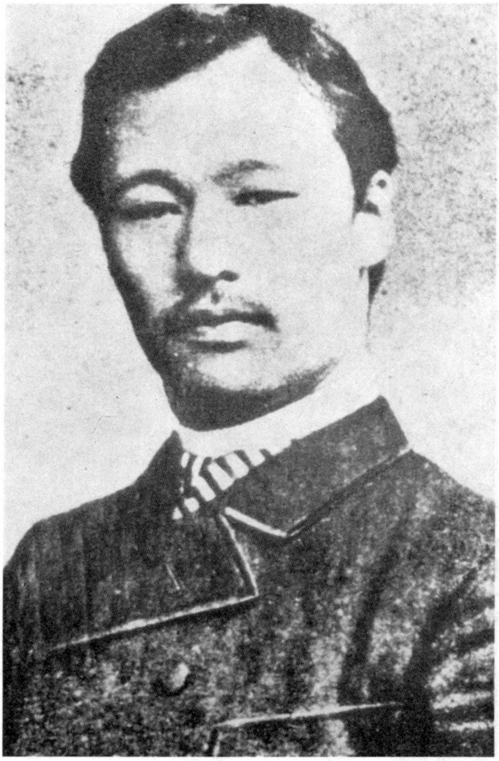

Fig. 7. Rintaro Mori as Ogai Mori (1863–1922)

Pediatrics was introduced as an independent subject in 1889 by Tsukada Hirota (1860–1928), who had studied in Strasbourg. Three Japanese guest physicians worked at the Kaiserin-Auguste-Victoria-Hospital, which had opened in 1909.

In 1896 X-rays were discovered, and 2 years later the first X-ray apparatus was installed in a Tokyo hospital by Siemens. A German textbook on radiology was translated into Japanese in 1914.

The outbreak of the First World War marked the end of this fruitful period of teamwork for the scientists of both countries. The Japanese left Germany. After the war economic hardship prevailed in all walks of life. Moreover, German scientists were forced into isolation. Attempts were made by both countries to renew the old contacts, and Ambassador Wilhelm Solf (1862–1936), who was sent to Japan in 1920, was a good intermediary. In the same year messages from individual Japanese scientists reached Germany, aimed "against the boycott of German scholars and doctors." Financial support also came from the president of the Japanese pharmaceutical company, Hajime Hoshi, as well as donations for the Kaiserin-Auguste-Victoria-Hospital, without which "the clinic would have had to close its doors in the years 1922–1923". In 1923 Japanese scientists and the Japanese Society of Radiologists collected money to save the Chair of Physics at the University of Würzburg.

Invitations from Japanese scientists to their German colleagues were an even greater expression of their attachment than the financial support. Here mention should be made of Aihiko Sata in Osaka who founded the Japanese–German Society Osaka-Kobe-Kyoto in 1920, and in connection with this a Japanese–German Institute. Other supporters were Baron Shinpei Goto (born 1857–1929), Tatsukichi Irisawa (1865–1939) and Nagayoshi Nagai (1845–1929), who had worked in Germany as young medical scientists before 1900. In 1922 Albert Einstein (1879–1955) accepted an invitation to give a lecture tour in Japan. During the voyage there he received the news that he had been awarded the Nobel Prize. On the ship he made the acquaintance of the surgeon Hayasi Miyake. This was the beginning of the friendship between the two but they did not see each other again: Einstein left Germany in 1933 and Miyake did not arrive in Kiel until 1934. Ludwig Aschoff and Fritz Haber accepted invitations to Japan in 1924. From 1922 to 1930, Fritz Härtel (1880–1940) (Fig. 8) from Berlin was Professor of Surgery at the University of Osaka. Mikio Ozawa first acted as his interpreter, then as his assistant, later as his senior physician, and in 1930 became his successor. During his 8 years of service, Härtel had trained 63 physicians as specialists in surgery. More than 1200 students attended his lectures. They dedicated a book, *Professor Fritz Härtel in Japan*, to his memory.

In the mid-1920s, relations between the Japanese and the Germans had returned to normal in the field of medicine. The establishment of a German–Japanese institute in Berlin and a Japanese–German cultural institute in Tokyo in 1926 were evidence of this. This had been preceded in 1925 by the foundation of the German Academic Exchange Service (DAAD) and the Alexander-von-Humboldt-Stiftung in Berlin. In 1934, Japan and Germany agreed to exchange students and young scientists. On the German side, grants were provided by the DAAD. In 1936 an agreement to establish a Japanese-German medical society in the Kaiserin Friedrich House in Berlin was signed by the Reichsärzteführer,

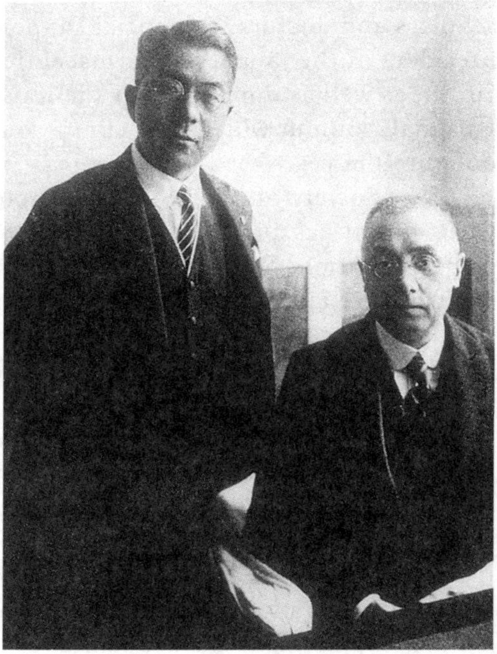

Fig. 8. Fritz Härtel (1880–1940) and Mikio Ozawa

Dr. Gerhard Wagner, and the Imperial Japanese Ambassador, Viscount Kinmoto Mushamokoji. In the years which followed, many visits took place; German army medical officers, for example, went to Japan and in 1938 the president of the Japanese–German Medical Society, Choei Ishibashi, came to Germany. In 1939, the war put an end to these contacts. Only one further exchange of ten Japanese and seven German students took place, in 1941.

After the military defeat in 1945, the American occupying forces introduced their medical school system to Japan. Memories of the ties with Germany, which had grown over five decades, still remained alive, however. In 1950, the DAAD and the Alexander-von-Humboldt-Stiftung, now independent institutions, were re-founded with their headquarters in Bonn. In 1952, after the resumption of diplomatic relations and the reopening of the Japanese–German Society in Tokyo, the first scholarship-holders arrived in Germany. In the report of the Alexander-von-Humboldt-Stiftung's work for a period of 30 years (1953–1983) the following figures are to be found with regard to Japan and medicine: 309 scholarship-holders, of whom almost 25% were from the medical profession. During the same period, of 176 scholarship-holders at the Free University, Berlin, 34 were from the field of medicine.

A new form of exchange, which brought scientists from both countries together, consisted of lecture tours and conferences. As early as 1957 Ishibashi came regularly to the Therapy Week in Karlsruhe and to visit Lüschke, the medical director of the Kaiserin-Auguste-Victoria-Hospital, who was a personal friend of his. In 1964 the Ishibashi Scholarship was set up at the Free University to enable "a Japanese physician to continue his training in pediatrics for one year". The scholarship was awarded until 1970. In 1963 Oshima came to Germany to introduce the gastrocamera. He stayed for 10 years, working for the first three in Erlangen, the rest at the Free University, Berlin. In Munich in 1965 he presented the combined gastrocamera and fibroscope, which had since been developed in Japan. In 1972 he wrote in the journal *Aktuelle Gastroenterologie* that, since 1968, West Germany with West Berlin had been the leading country among those possessing this apparatus.

Since then many medical meetings and congresses have been organized in Germany or in Japan with participants from both countries. In the field of surgery, the Japanese–German Surgical Association was founded in 1994.

CHAPTER 13

The Relationship Between Japan and Germany in Medicine: Mutual Stimulation

E. DELTZ

Reflections on mutual relationships between German medical sciences and theoretical and practical medicine in Japan go far beyond the limits of medical history. They offer a view of a fascinating interplay between two cultures in which there are various mutual political and pragmatic influences as well as scientific and intellectual aspects.

In the relationship between Japanese and German medicine (regarded as part of European medicine) three main epochs can be distinguished.

1. The phase of limited contact of Japanese with Dutch-German medicine during the Azuchi-Momoyama (1569–1615) and Edo (1616–1867) periods
2. The adoption of German medical sciences after the isolation of Japan ended in the Meiji era (from 1868)
3. The time after the beginning of the twentieth century, when Japan came in direct contact with Germany through its own scientific contributions after it had established a western-orientated medical system

Chinese medicine was introduced to Japan during the Heian period (784–1186) [4]. The Chinese had created a complete though speculative system of the human body in which the organs were considered to be connected by a system of vessels through which blood and "pneuma" could circulate. Physiology was influenced by the dual principle of male (positive) and female (negative) [4]. During the Kamakura period (1187–1333) compilations of Chinese medical manuscripts were assembled.

The Muromachi period (1334–1568) and the Azuchi-Momoyama era that followed (1569–1615) were characterized by both civil wars and radical political changes. It was a period of stagnancy in scientific development. During this decisive period in

Japanese history Christianity, together with European sciences and medicine, was brought to Japan by Portuguese missionaries . In this way the fascinating contact between two cultures began, with mutual influence and fertilization.

The Portuguese, who were called *Nanbanjin*, i.e. "southern barbarians", were seen for the first time on the island of Kyushu. A lively communication developed between them and the Japanese. The knowledge brought from Europe to Japan by the Portuguese was called the "science of the southern barbarians" (*Nanbangaku*), thus becoming the precursor of what was later called Dutch science (*Rangaku*) [1].

The physicians and surgeons who worked amongst the Portuguese missionaries developed intensive teaching activities. Through this they became the founders of *Nanban Ryu-Geka* i.e. the surgery of the school of southern barbarians. The first contacts between occidental and Japanese medicine had been established.

In 1585 Christianity in Japan was prohibited by Hideyoshi Toyotomi and all missionaries and therefore also all foreign doctors were expelled from the country. In 1597 the Dutch appeared on the west coast of Kyushu and obtained permission for free trade. In this way the Dutch took over an important role as mediators between western culture and Japan during the complete isolation of the country (*Sakoku*) which was to last more than 200 years.

Through the activities of the East India Trading Company several kinds of goods, especially drugs, were imported into Japan. In contrast, importing books into Japan was strictly forbidden. The *Oranda Tsuji*, as the Japanese interpreters who worked at the Dutch trading post on the island of Dejima were called, were however allowed to be in contact with the Dutch physicians to gain medical knowledge from them. The first Germans came to Japan through these Dutch trade connections [8].

The first German traveller to reach Japan was Michael Hohreiter from Ulm. He visited Japan during his journey-through East Asia in 1618. In 1683 or 1684 the barber and surgeon Christoph Fink had the opportunity to visit Dejima. Several other German travellers brought information about Japan to Germany and Europe at the end of seventeenth century, contributing to knowledge about this distant and mysterious country.

A comprehensive compilation of contemporary knowledge of Japan was produced by Bernhard Varen (born in 1622 in Hitzacker, died 1650 in Amsterdam) with his important work *Descriptio regni japoniae*. So during the seventeenth century an image of Japan emerged in Middle Europe which had certain features in regard to geography, daily life, and fauna and flora.

In the area of medicine contacts became closer. The first physician who worked at the trade post of Dejima was the German Caspar S. Schamberger who stayed in Japan in 1641 or 1649. He founded the *Kaspar-Ryu-Geka*, i.e. the Kaspar School of Surgery. He and his successors Hoffmann, Katz, Palm, Striefen and Ten Rhyne during their stay in Dejima taught European medicine to the Japanese interpreters. After some of these interpreters had gained some insight into European medicine, they were declared to be doctors. After that they used to add to their names *Oranda Ryu Geka*, i.e. surgery according to the Dutch medical school.

On 9 September 1690 the physician Engelbert Kaempfer reached Japan during his employment by the Dutch East India Trading Company. In 1691 and 1692 he joined the head of the trading post of Dejima (Opperhooft) in his annual journey (Hofreis) to the imperial court in Edo. Besides his medical activities Kaempfer was committed to a comprehensive investigation of Japan. His main interests were in the field of botany.

The results of his work, which he brought back to Germany in 1683, could not be published until 1712, when his work *Amoenitum exoticarum politico-physico-medicarum* appeared. As Kaempfer died in 1716 he was unable to publish his main work, *Japan in Our Time*, himself.

Kaempfer's studies not only resulted in an exact and extensive description of the country but also laid the foundations for a better assessment of religious and political conditions and for contemporary European ideas about Japan to be corrected. He understood that the isolation of the country ordered by the shogunate was not only a measure to avoid subjugation by European nations but also an opportunity for Japan to create its own culture, which led Japan to "a summit of blissful state" [8].

Kaempfer tried to obtain information about Japanese medicine. In his *Amoenitates exoticae* (Lemgo 1712) there are reports about acupuncture and moxibustion and about the history of tea, which was used as a medicine in Japan. Although he left various handwritten records about Japanese medicine Kaempfer did not succeed in transferring his special knowledge to the European public. He was also unable to understand and describe the traditional roots and philosophical background of Japanese medicine. In addition, the strange techniques of acupuncture and moxibustion were not accepted by the scientific authorities of the eighteenth century. The impact of Kaempfer's knowledge of Japanese medicine was therefore extremely limited in Europe [6]. The main purpose of his journeys, observations and publications was to explore the country of Japan, not to impart his knowledge of medicine.

At that time fundamental changes took place in the medical history of Japan. These led to a gradual turning away from philosophically based Chinese medicine and a transition to medical sciences founded on the empirical principles of natural science which had proved to be a workable foundation for western medicine. The theories of Chinese medicine are part of the Confucian concept of the world as a harmonious universe. This philosophical system was in contrast to the European concept of the medical sciences as transported to Japan by its Dutch-German contacts. The European concept was mainly based on empirical experience in the observation and treatment of disease and followed the theoretical concepts of Wilhelm Hufeland (1762–1836) [2]. His works, which were translated into Japanese, had a considerable influence in Japan [13]. Essential contributions to medical ideas at that time were made by the school of Vienna (van Swieten), which originated from the Leiden school of medicine (Hermann Boerhaave).

The work of the surgeon Lorenz Heister (1683–1758) from Frankfurt was translated by Gempaku Sugita (1733–1817). The *Compendium institionum chirurgicum* by Joseph Jakob von Plenck (1733–1807) became the first systematic textbook of surgery in Japan [13]. Heister's works were well known in the Dutch translation entitled *Heelkundige Onderwijizingen.*

Because the theories of European science were not well known in Japan, these medical facts and opinions could only be adapted by the Japanese without consideration of the theoretical background. Discourse on anatomy in Japan is a good example of the scientific confrontation which arose from the new scientific findings brought to Japan from Europe. The Confucian doctrine which teaches the inviolability of the human body, as well as the

Buddhist reverence for the dead, had prevented scientific investigation of the human body. Therefore the first systematic autopsy in Japan was not done until 1754. Toyo Yamawaki (1705–1762), who was present at this event, then became convinced that traditional Chinese anatomical works were wrong. He was therefore induced to write the treatise *Zoshi* (i.e. description of internal organs) [4, 7]. This book, the first original work on anatomy in Japan, was rejected by the followers of the traditional school. This denial however could not prevent subsequent autopsies and the comparison of anatomical findings with European anatomical works. The results were more exact anatomical textbooks, e.g. *Kaishihen* (on the understanding of the body) by Motoyoshi Ogino (1737–1806) and Nobuto Kawaguchi (1736–1811).

Among the books brought to Japan by the Dutch traders was a beginners' textbook on anatomy. It was the Dutch translation by Gerard Dicten of a work by Johann Adam Kulmus which appeared in Amsterdam in 1734. Kulmus was born in Breslau and had been a member of the Academy of Science in Berlin since 1725 [5, 13]. This Dutch translation of Kulmus's anatomical tables (*Tabulae anatomicae in quibus corporis humani*, 1722) made it possible for Ryotaku Maeno (1723–1803) and Sugita Gempaku to assess the findings they made during a post-mortem examination of an executed woman in 1771. Both authors were astonished and impressed by the accuracy of this western work, to such an extent that, with Nakakawa Jun`an (1739–1780), they were persuaded to produce a translation which was published after 3 years and 5 months' work as *Kaitai Shinsho* ("New text on dissection-anatomy") in 1774 [4, 5, 13]. Publication of this epochal work was not just a decisive point in the development of Japanese medicine, as there now existed a basic anatomic work which was orientated towards western scientific criteria, but also marked the beginning of so-called Dutch studies (*Rangaku*) [5, 11].

In his *Rangaku-Kotohajime* (beginning of Dutch studies) published in 1815 Sugita Gempaku stressed the significance of the translation work which was the forerunner of *Kaitai Shinsho* in introducing western science to Japan. He pointed out that he and his coworkers had created the expression *Rangaku* in 1794 after publishing the *Kaitai Shinsho* [5]. This work is therefore an important bridge between European and Japanese science. It not only established the fundamentals of anatomy in Japan but also introduced an integrated view of Japanese work and European scientific work originally written in Latin, English, German or French and then translated into Dutch. These translated works had been translated into Japanese by the *Rangaku sha* (scholars of Dutch studies), thus forming the basis of Japanese scientific development. *Rangaku* started by dealing with medical works but soon included other disciplines and from the beginning of the nineteenth century it developed into science in the western sense [5, 11].

It was this scientific landscape into which the last and most important German physician and scientist – Philipp Franz von Siebold – entered. His life and work have already been dealt with in several contributions to this volume. In his main work *Nippon* and in his *Atlas and nautical charts of the Japanese empire* Siebold presented abundant new knowledge of Japan. With these books he significantly advanced geographic and especially ethnographic studies in Europe. His collections brought to Europe from Japan served as a basis for the ethnographic museum in Leiden, which was a model for ethnographic museums in Paris, Copenhagen and Munich.

The physicians Kaempfer and Siebold influenced the European world of thought by collecting, analyzing and distributing knowledge about Japan. The main direction of their activities was from Japan towards Europe.

The adoption of German and other European sources of scientific data was extended from *Rangaku,* studies based on Dutch translations, to other western sciences (*Yogaku*), in which books from different European countries were analyzed. These books were catalogued in the examining institute for foreign writings (*Bansho shirabesho*) which was founded in 1856 and later became part of the University of Tokyo (11).

The study of European-German medicine and other sciences was not however characterized by any systematic and methodical intellectual exchange. The contact with European sciences primarily had the merely pragmatic goal of assimilating economic and medical knowledge [5]. As physicians for the Dutch trading post of Dejima were selected only on the basis of their usefulness in aspects of practical medicine, these doctors could not serve as scientifically qualified teachers of medical sciences for the Japanese [5].

Even though *Rangaku* expanded to include studies of different sciences derived from Europe, the approach to German medical sources did not fundamentally change until the Meiji restoration began. In one of the edicts of the Imperial Proclamation of 6 April 1868 "striving for knowledge of the whole world" was particularly emphasized. [14].

These efforts to adapt scientific knowledge from different countries of the world symbolize a fundamental change in the attitude of mind as well as in scientific theories which took place in the middle of the nineteenth century. The result of this drastic change was the introduction of German medicine to Japan [13, 14].

The reasons for the change were threefold [13, 14]. The Japanese had recognized that many of the medical textbooks, including Kulmus's anatomic tables, had been decisive in the creation of *Kaitai Shinsho* and the origin of *Rangaku* therefore lay in German sources. The second reason was the dominant influence of Philipp Franz von Siebold as a representative of German medicine. The deciding factor obviously was that Japan had come to realize that German medicine at the beginning of the second half of the nineteenth century held a leading position.

At that time various eminent clinicians and theoretical medical scientists were working in Germany, e.g. the physiologist Johannes Müller (1801–1858), the internist Johannes Lukas Schönlein (1793–1864) and the anatomists Theodor Schwann (1810–1885) and Jacob Henle (1809–1885). Rudolf Virchow (1821–1902) had laid the fundamentals of modern pathological anatomy by his basic theory of cellular pathology. In the field of surgery Richard von Volkmann (1830–1889) and Theodor Billroth (1829–1894) had expanded the methods of surgical treatment and had laid the fundamentals of clinical research in surgery.

The second period of the interchange in medical science between Germany and Japan began at the beginning of the Meiji era (1868) and was characterized by the adoption of German medical sciences (see Chap. 12, this volume).

The first German medical doctors to work in Japan were the surgeon Leopold Müller (1822–1893) and the internist Theodor Hoffmann (1837–1894), who arrived in Yokohama on 23 August 1871. They immediately began to introduce a system of medical education orientated towards German university training [13, 14].

The successor to Müller was Emil-August-Wilhelm Schulze, who had been educated by von Bardeleben at the Charité in Berlin. He made a great contribution to the introduction of antisepsis into Japan, which he had learned from Lister. He gave a vivid description of his professional and personal experiences in his letters to Germany, published in 1980 [10].

Hoffmann's successor was Agaton Wernich, who was followed by Erwin Otto Baelz (1849–1913), who became the best known and most important of German medical teachers in Japan [12]. Besides his activities as an academic teacher in Tokyo Baelz wrote more than 60 scientific papers which dealt mainly with that infectious diseases occurring in Japan, such as leprosy, cholera and typhus. He first described *Tsutsugamushi,* or flood fever; he also discovered the pulmonary leech (*Diostoma pulmonale*) and described the effects of hot springs and many other ethnographic subjects. His successful medical activities gave him such an outstanding reputation that he was appointed personal physician to the imperial family. In 1889 the title *Shokunin* was conferred on him, which was the highest rank a foreigner in the service of the Japanese government could receive.

The surgeon who worked with Baelz in Tokyo was Julius Scriba, who was famous for his outstanding surgical skill. In 1888 he performed the first nephrectomy in Japan and he did pioneering work in the field of surgery of the stomach [12]. His instructions on war surgery were particularly appreciated by Japanese surgeons who benefited from such knowledge during the Russo-Japanese war (1905).

Erwin Baelz became an authority in medicine whose domain extended far beyond Japan. In addition he had become a critical observer of the radical changes in eastern Asia at the turn of the country. In letters and publications he examined the problematic relations between European countries, especially Germany, and the developing great powers, China and Japan. The German government at that time failed to make use of Baelz's profound knowledge of Japan. He was then very concerned to realize that anti German opinion was gradually increasing in Japan. He was critical of the German ambassadors in Japan, Gutschmidt and Counts Leyden and Wede, whose actions were characterized by a complete lack of empathy with and a low opinion of the Japanese. The gradually developing tensions between Germany and Japan plunged him into despair as his life's work had been for the benefit of Japan. By his various activities Baelz had laid the essential basis for the development of modern medicine in Japan, especially for the development of the Imperial University in Tokyo.

As this university developed, German academic teachers were gradually replaced by Japanese professors. So more and more original Japanese scientists and physicians appeared who had a formative influence on medical science in Japan.

By this time the third and last period of the relationship between Japan and Germany in medicine had begun: this was after the turn of the century, when with the establishment of a western medical system in Japan Japanese doctors were able to contribute to medical research with genuinely scientific work.

Many of the Japanese doctors who had been educated by German teachers continued their studies in Germany. In particular, several Japanese scientists worked with Robert Koch (1843–1901), Emil von Behring (1854–1917), and Paul Ehrlich (1854–1915).

One of Baelz's students was Shibasoburu Kitasato (1856–1931) who came to Germany in 1885 and became an assistant to Robert Koch. Together they succeeded in preparing pure cultures of tetanus bacilli. This opened a completely new epoch of serum therapy which created the possibility of defeating diphtheria and tetanus. In 1890 Kitasato published a paper with Emil von Behring entitled "Über das Zustandekommen der Diphterie-immunität und der Tetanusimmunität bei Tieren". This work was the basis for the production of tetanus and diphtheria serum, and von Behring was awarded the Nobel Prize for his scientific contributions [3].

One of Kitasato's most important pupils was Sahachiro Hata (1873–1938). Hata became world-famous as a co-worker of Paul Ehrlich (1854–1915). Ehrlich had created the fundamentals of chemotherapy with the basic idea that the affinity of a chemical agent to the protoplasm of living cells consisted in a specific interaction of the molecules of chemical substances with the side chains of the cells ("Seitenkettentheorie"). A decisive success was the development of the agent dioxidiaminobenzoate which proved to be effective against spirochetes, thus creating the first substance which could cure syphilis. This drug was at first called Ehrlich-Hata 606 and later became famous as Salvarsan.

Other famous Japanese scientists who worked in Germany included Kiyoshi Shiga (1870–1957), who in 1898 discovered the bacterium named after him that causes dysentery, and Tawara Subaro, who with the pathologist Ludwig Aschoff (1866–1942) in Freiburg described the excitation-conduction system of the heart.

During these collaborations in scientific projects, fruitful scientific and personal contacts developed between German and Japanese scientists, leading to relationships between teachers and pupils which lasted for decades. An impressive example is the report of the cooperation of Kitasato and Robert Koch [9].

From about the time of the First World War Japanese medicine gained independence from Germany. The last close contact with Japan that resembled the contacts of the nineteenth century was with Fritz Härtel, a surgeon from Halle who worked as a surgical teacher in Osaka and was involved in the building of the surgical university hospital there. Simultaneously closer cooperation with England and the United States began.

In the course of the general deterioration of international relations after the Second World War contact between German scientists and their Japanese colleagues was naturally reduced. But the former good relationship between Japan and Germany has gradually been reactivated so that personal and scientific contacts can still develop today.

Japanese researchers made important contributions in the field of endoscopy which had been opened in 1868 by Kussmaul, who used the first rigid gastroscope. After the development of semiflexible endoscopes in the 1930s and 1940s Hirschowitz introduced the first flexible gastroscope, which was paralleled by the development of the blind gastrocamera by Uji. Japanese companies made significant contributions to the further development of endoscope technology.

Closely connected with the work of Japanese endoscopists is the research of Japanese surgeons in the field of gastric and lung cancer. Important investigations especially in regard to lymphatic drainage of the stomach and bronchi have been made recently.

In summary, the mutual interconnections between German and Japanese medicine started with indirect mediation via Dutch contacts with Japan. Intensive research activities by Engelbert Kaempfer and Philipp Franz von Siebold established the first scientific exchanges. This consisted mainly of ethnographic, botanical and zoological studies and was in principle directed from Japan to Europe. *Rangaku* studies were the vehicle for transporting medical knowledge from Germany to Japan, albeit not in a systematic manner.

Systematic transfer of medical knowledge started with the Meiji restoration at the beginning of the 1870s. In this way, since the end of the nineteenth century the fundamentals have been laid for genuinely creative development in the medical sciences, thus making Japan nowadays one of the leading nations in medical research and health care.

References

1. Dettmer HA (1987) Einführung in das Studium der japanischen Geschichte. Wissenschaftliche Buchgesellschaft, Darmstadt
2. Diepgen P (1919) Geschichte der Medizin. Göschen, Berlin
3. Eckart W (1994) Geschichte der Medizin. Springer, Berlin Heidelberg New York
4. Fujikawa J (1976) Der Arzt in der japanischen Kultur. Robugen, Esslingen
5. Goodman G (1984) Dutch studies in Japan re-examined. In: Kreiner J (ed) Deutschland–Japan, historische Kontakte. Bouvier/Grundmann, Bonn
6. Haberlandt D (1993) Zwischen Wunderkammer und Forschungsbericht – Engelbert Kaempfers Beitrag zum europäischen Japanbild in Japan und Europa, 1543–1929. In: Croissant D, Ledderhose L (eds) Berliner Festspiele. Argon, Berlin
7. Johei S (1993) Vom Sinnbild zum Abbild. Malerei und Naturwissenschaften in der Edo-Zeit in Japan und Europa, 1543–1929. In: Croissant D, Ledderhose L (eds) Berliner Festspiele. Argon, Berlin
8. Kreiner J (1984) Deutschland–Japan, die frühen Jahrhunderte. In: Kreiner J (ed) Deutschland–Japan, historische Kontakte. Bouvier/Grundmann, Bonn
9. Mijajima M (1935) Lehrer und Schüler. z, Tokyo
10. Schulze W (1980) Ein deutscher Chirurg und seine Frau in Japan vor hundert Jahren. Briefe. In: Hesekiel T (ed) z, Lübeck
11. Tadashi Y (1993) Rangaku – die holländischen Wissenschaften in Japan und Europa, 1543–1929. In: Croissant D, Ledderhose L (eds) Berliner Festspiele. Argon, Berlin
12. Versovi G (1972) Erwin Baelz, Wegbereiter der japanischen Medizin. Schriftenreihe der Bezirksärztekammer Nordwürttemberg Nr. 22. Gentner, Stuttgart

13. Vianden H-H (1985) Die Einführung der deutschen Medizin im Japan der Meiji-Zeit. In: Schadewald H (ed) Düsseldorfer Arbeit zur Geschichte der Medizin. Trieltsch, Düsseldorf
14. Yasumasa O (1993) Die Malerei im westlichen Stil in der Edo-Zeit in Japan und Europa, 1543–1929. In: Croissant D, Ledderhose L (eds) Berliner Festspiele. Argon, Berlin

History, Present State and Future Perspectives of European–Japanese Cooperation in Culture, Economy and Science

J. KREINER

Engelbert Kaempfer of Lemgo in Westphalia, Philipp Franz von Siebold of Würzburg, and Erwin von Baelz of Bietigheim in Swabia: three names that come up almost without fail at any official event promoting German–Japanese relations. They personify the history of Euro-Japanese contact and the German part in it, the acquisition of knowledge about Japan by Europeans, the growth of Japanese studies, and the rise of modern natural sciences – particularly medicine – in Japan.

We could extend the list at will. Caspar Schamberger of Leipzig was a long-standing adviser to the court physicians of the third shogun, Iemitsu, as early as the mid-seventeenth century. It is to him that Japan owes its oldest school of surgery, *Kasuparu-ryû-geka*. Andreas Cleyer of Kassel, a trained apothecary and in 1682–83 and 1685–86 twice *opperhoofd* (in Japanese *kapitan*) of the Dutch trading post on Dejima in Nagasaki Bay, founded through botanical research with his gardener, Georg Meister of Saxony, a major branch of Japanese studies that extended into the nineteenth century by way of Kaempfer, Carl Peter Thunberg and Siebold. After 1868, there followed numerous individuals who significantly contributed not only to our knowledge about Japan, but also to the rise in Japan of modern science, administration and western lifestyles. It would be unfair to single out any one such individual here.

We should be aware that contacts with Japan, beginning with the first encounter on the island of Tanega in 1543, were always fully European. Admittedly, it was the Spanish and the Portuguese who went out and forged the first links in the sixteenth century, to be joined by the British for a brief period during the early seventeenth century. And for more than 200 years, from 1641 to the "opening" of the country in 1853/54, the sole trading post in Japan was Dutch. Yet none of these enterprises was a one-nation affair. All were wholly and severally European: the Spanish crown was united with that of the Holy Roman Empire under a Habsburg, Carlo I of Spain/Charles V of Austria; Philip II of Spain granted the monopoly over East Asian and Japanese trade to the Fugger family of Augsburg; despite their southern European roots, the Jesuit and Franciscan orders included friars from north of the Alps; and the Dutch East India Company drew its recruits from all corners of Europe. In the eighteenth century, for which there are complete hiring lists, about one third of all voyagers to the East Indies and Japan came from Germany, Scandinavia, the Baltic and Scotland; that is, from the economically backward areas of Europe. Most of the Germans came from the southwest of the country.

Nonetheless, most scientific exchange with Japan was driven by the Dutch themselves, and this despite the fierce criticism they elicited for their alleged profiteering in Europe. I refer the reader to Jonathan Swift's *Gulliver's Travels* (1726), Oliver Goldsmith's *Letters from a Chinese Philosopher Residing in London to his Friends in the East* (1762), and Adam Johann von Krusenstern's *Voyage Round the World in the Years 1803, 1804, 1805 and 1806 (1810/11)*. Krusenstern expressly states, "This [the Dutch] nation Europe owes nothing for its knowledge of the Japanese Empire". On the contrary, *opperhoofd* Isaac Titsingh (Dejima, 1779/80 and 1782/84) collected folklore, books and maps. In 1819 and 1822, he published two seminal reference works, *Cerémonies usitées au Japon* ..." and *Illustrations of Japan*. His successors, Hendrik Doeff and Jan Cock Blomhoff (*opperhoofd* 1803–1817 and 1817–1823, respectively), aided mutual understanding through the *Haruma-wage* Dutch–Japanese dictionary (Doeff) and a comprehensive collection of Japanese objects (Blomhoff). Siebold would have been unable to open his surgery in Narutaki without Blomhoff's help as an intermediary. Siebold also learned much from Blomhoff's collection, and took many items for his own collection from those of Blomhoff and Johann Frederic van Overmeer-Fisscher.

There is another point that we should not overlook: At no time did Japan consider itself a "closed country". Early seventeenth-century geopolitical events – the union of the Spanish and Portuguese crowns, the Spanish occupation of the Philippines, the establishment of a sea link between Manila and Acapulco, the fall of the Ming Dynasty, and the siege of Taiwan led by Admiral

Coxinga (Zheng Chenggong) – gave Japan grounds to rethink its past expansionist policy. The suspicion was reinforced by domestic structural reforms. A number of decrees restricted foreign dealings, though there was never a blanket ban: Dutch, English, Chinese and Koreans alike could come and go as they pleased. The idea that Japan was "closed" came only later, when Kaempfer summed up Japanese policy as a plan "to shut up the country" and praised this – along with many European thinkers, including Kant, Fichte, Matthias Claudius, and the Hegelian Karl Rosenkranz – as worthy of emulation. Nor did the concept become known (as *sakoku*) to the Japanese until the relevant passage of Kaempfer's *The History of Japan* (1727) was translated in 1811. It underlies both our understanding of Japan and Japan's understanding of its own history to this day.

This in principle open, if selective, policy towards foreign contact also prevented Japan from falling behind Europe in development. Indeed, its history has run an astoundingly parallel course, as many historians have been eager to point out, and as President Roman Herzog reiterated on his spring 1997 state visit to Japan. Thus, from the Kamakura period onwards, Japan's history largely mirrors European feudalism. In the wake of overseas trade and Japanese voyages of discovery, the sixteenth century saw the emergence of trading ports, such as Hakata and Sakai, comparable to the Free Cities of the Holy Roman Empire. From 1600, the Edo period saw the rise of a merchant class with its own distinctive culture, a culture which strongly influences that of Europe today – for example in theater, architecture and design.

Neo-Confucianism, which largely owed its propagation as a state ideology to the fifth Tokugawa shogun, Tsunayoshi (1680–1709), was tagged an "Enlightenment" and publicized as such in Europe by as early a figure as Kaempfer. This ideology nurtured the growth of experimental scientific research in Japan, research that was additionally able to profit from the high technology of the time. To Europeans of the seventeenth and early eighteenth century, Japan thus seemed at least an equal – if not a model – in both intellectual endeavor and the natural sciences. The same Georg Meister mentioned earlier sums up this attitude best in his *Der Orientalisch-Indianische Kunst- und Lust-Gärtner* of 1692: As Japan "needs no European ... as mentor in matters of art, science or worldly venture ..., whence no European may delude himself that we alone be wise ..., and if there exists under the sun a people of wise conduct [and] sound principles in state governance and commerce alike ..., then it is in all truth the Japanese."

This tradition provided fertile soil for rapid adoption and refinement of the knowledge of European advances in the natural sciences imparted by way of the *Rangaku* or "Dutch sciences". And the Japanese were well able to choose wisely among the proffered treats: When at Edo in the late 1650s a physician accompanying *opperhoofd* Zacharias Wagner prepared an ointment of fox fat that stank out the entire quarters of the Dutch delegation, the Japanese colleagues present were suitably unimpressed. The same fate befell Engelbert Kaempfer with the wound-dressing plaster he described to the shogun's court physicians. The surgeons, on the other hand, fared better – from Caspar Schamberger through to Philipp Franz von Siebold. As recently as the late nineteenth century, Erwin Baelz owed his success not so much to internal medicine, but to the field of hygiene and nutritional science that was so crucial to the army (and for whose study the army had originally sent staff surgeon Ogai Mori to Germany).

While Japan had thus acquired a fairly accurate picture of Europe by the mid-nineteenth century, the Enlightenment and ensuing Eurocentrism in particular had profoundly changed European notions of Japan for the worse. The universal high regard of Japan as a model was displaced by contempt. In a 1776 letter to Voltaire, Frederick the Great of Prussia wrote that since political decisions were taken in Europe, knowledge of Japan was a mere "curiosity". Christoph Meiners, a historian from Göttingen, went even further in a pamphlet of 1790 ("Über die Natur der Völker im südlichen Asien, auf den Ostindischen und Südsee-Inseln und in den Südländern"). In it, he ascribes Japan and all "Altaic peoples" a "complete lack of inventiveness and of scientific spirit". Accordingly, Japan can "only copy, and cannot invent". This opinion was widely adopted and, regrettably, persists to this day.

This view was compounded by Japan's readiness to glorify Europe as a model for its own modernization, starting (with the Meiji Restoration) in 1868. The high-ranking Iwakura mission to America and Europe of 1871–1873 was influential in this regard. The German Empire in particular lent itself as a model for Japan, the two having become modern nation states at more or less the same time (the 1868 Meiji Restoration, 1871 abdication of feudal lords and 1879 annexation of the Kingdom of Ryûkyû in Japan paralleling the founding of the German Empire in 1871; similarly Italian unification in 1870 and the Austro-Hungarian *Ausgleich* of 1867).

Japan realized that the "lead" gained by the great European powers, though slight, might suffice to jeopardize its continued existence as an independent state and its later acceptance as an equal. In response, it brought in large numbers of European scientists and scholars along with administrators and the like as advisors. On the one hand, it was the presence of these advisors that first popularized the view in Japan itself that it must catch up and "learn from Europe". On the other, it boosted European self-assurance to the point of self-conceit: on returning home, many of the "teachers" spoke of the Japanese as "pupils", or even "children". The quarrel between the geologist Edmund Naumann and Mori Ogai, fought out in the pages of the *Augsburger Allgemeine Zeitung* (1886/87), was but one witness of this trend.

To summarize so far, we should be aware that by about 1900, foreign stereotypes had arisen in Europe (including Germany) and Japan that bore no relation to the 300-year history of contact, or indeed to reality. Yet they influence our notions of each other to this day, often subconsciously. The foregoing detailed historical introduction is thus necessary to a better understanding of the present.

Full scale industrialization, military victories against China in 1894/95 and the European power Russia in 1905, and above all the alliance with Great Britain of 1902 at first gave rise to the feeling in Japan that it had now completed the tasks set by its European mentors – most of whom had been replaced by their Japanese protégés on retiring from service (which Baelz and many others did only with great reluctance). But two other events then made clear to Japan that, for all its progress, it would continue to need western civilization and science as a model for the time being: Although Japan attended the Versailles peace negotiations as a victorious power, its demand for a clause in the League of Nations Covenant proscribing racial discrimination was denied. Yet more important to science was the "Einstein shock" of 1922.

Out of allegiance and gratitude towards German scientists, and doubtless also for fear of now joining the "have-nots" togehter with Germany, Japan became the first nation to break the boycott on German science after the First World War, by inviting Albert Einstein to lecture on his theory of relativity. It was at this very time that Einstein received the Nobel Prize, making Japan very aware of just how much remained to be done in the field of basic research. Accordingly, a group of people met in Tokyo to promote cooperation with Germany. Their patron was the pharmacist and industrialist Hajime Hoshi, who had married the daughter of the Strasbourg-trained anthropologist and student of Baelz, Yoshikiyo Koganei. The political side was represented by Goto Shinpei, who had done his M.D. under Pettenkofer at Munich, and Germany was represented by Ambassador Wilhelm Solf, an orientalist, expert on Buddhism, and bridge-builder between the two nations. A foundation was set up which made substantial funds available to the Kaiser Wilhelm Society (today's Max Planck Society). This "Japan Committee" was managed among others by Fritz Haber, Max Planck and Otto Hahn. German atomic physics most likely owed much of its early success to this support.

A second invitee to Japan, Fritz Haber, became convinced that Japan would contribute significantly to the sciences, and particularly the natural sciences – an insight that had already existed in the eighteenth century but, as we have seen, had since fallen into obscurity. Haber thought it important to learn about and to understand Japan. He persuaded Hoshi to make a further donation and the Kaiser Wilhelm Society to found a Japan Institute in Berlin. This latter was active in the field of Japanese studies from 1926, initially under the directorship of Friedrich Trautz, and later under that of Solf. Its counterpart in Japan was the Japanese-German Cultural Institute of Tokyo, set up in 1927. Also founded in 1926, on the initiative of André Malraux and Keizo Shibuzawa (entrepreneur, Director of the Bank of Japan, patron and passionate amateur ethnologist), was the Maison Franco-Japonais in Tokyo, an institute likewise dedicated to wide-ranging scientific exchange between Europe (with the emphasis on France) and Japan.

Yet once these first two European institutes were in place, there were no further moves to supplement "Japanology", in the narrow sense of philology and the study of Japanese literature, with efforts to promote all sciences as they related to Japan, including the natural sciences and social and economic studies. In fact, the work of the Japan Institute in Berlin was gradually curtailed – reflecting the contempt in which the Third Reich held Japan despite all propaganda to the contrary. During the Second World War the Institute was of no consequence whatsoever.

In America, on the other hand, Japanese studies flourished and enjoyed a fully interdisciplinary approach. There, Japanese studies came to mean area studies and supplanted retrospective, classical studies with their stigma of Eurocentrism. Similarly in Britain the army's Japanese language school educated a new generation of specialists who brought a Japanese component to a whole array of general disciplines. The leading light here was the sociologist Ronald P. Dore, whose own survey-based research into urban society in Tokyo, the land reforms, the education system, Japanese management practices, and the like profoundly influenced not only western research, but also research in Japan itself. Lord Scarbrough's *Report of the Interdepartmental Commission of Enquiry on Oriental, Slavonic, East European and African Studies* of 1947 then set the stage for a redirection of Japanese studies in the UK. The report notes, with some levity, "Students of Far Eastern Languages ... tend to become like a man who is always taking his car to pieces and never goes for a drive. I have known many ... Japanologues who never lift their noses from their texts and consequently do not know what is going on in the Oriental world around them."

Accordingly, the subsequent Report of the Hayter Sub-Commission (1961) demanded "that development should take place not so much in the language sector as in the fields of history, geography, law, economics and other social science departments; secondly, that students outside the 'language departments' should be exposed to the ideas, the history and the problems of the non-western world [i.e. including Japan], and, thirdly, that a happier balance should be achieved between linguistic and non-linguistic studies and between classical and modern interests".

In response, a Centre for Japanese Studies was established at the University of Sheffield in 1963. More significant, however, was the restructuring of the University of London School of Oriental and African Studies (SOAS), founded in 1917 along the lines of the Seminar für Orientalische Sprachen in Berlin. The UK thus became the first European country to establish Japanese studies in a form that was appropriate to the times.

In the light of these efforts, it is understandable that even after large cuts in Japanese studies under Margaret Thatcher, a highly fruitful working relationship in all areas exists between the United Kingdom and Japan. This is further enhanced by substantial contributions from Japan, for example in the form of the

Nissan Institute in Oxford and the Suntory Chair at the London School of Economics. Moreover, such major events as the Japan Festival of 1981 followed in a long tradition of Japanese self-promotion that began in 1910 with the Great Japan-British Exhibition in London and reached its high point with the Great Japan Exhibition on Arts of the Edo Period in 1981.

No similar development was to be observed on the European continent for many years. Germany in particular lagged far behind both the USA and the UK. A revival of Japanology largely took place on the initiative of former teachers of German at Japanese colleges who had been forcibly repatriated after the war. For a long time, however, the focus remained on teaching the classical language of the pre-modern era and on textual study. Impulse for change came only from outside in the late 1960s, when the student protests of 1968 were sparked by the anachronistic syllabus of the Japanese Department at the Free University of Berlin and demanded a more contemporary course of study. At approximately the same time, the German government – along with German industry, startled at Japan's success – demanded explanations of how Japan had come to attain second place ahead of Germany in terms of gross national product. Traditional Japanology was unable to meet either demand. German universities responded during the 1970s by founding a number of Japanese studies departments and recruiting Japan experts from the social sciences. The Viennese School of ethnologist and Japanologist Alexander Slawik came to be held in particularly high regard. Today, approximately half of the 16 or so institutes of "Japanology" at German universities have a contemporary, social science-based curriculum with a vocational bias, including Bonn, Marburg, Tübingen and Trier. In contrast, Cologne, Frankfurt, Göttingen, Munich and Erlangen-Nürnberg remain primarily focused on the great tradition of Japanese literary and intellectual history. Bochum, Hamburg and the Free University of Berlin cover both sides. Where there was little hope for rapid change, the governing boards of some universities created an institute in parallel with the existing department of Japanology to gain a modern facility for Japanese studies, as with the Japan Center at the University of Munich. In the state of North Rhine-Westphalia particularly, the ministry responsible, in the person of the then Secretary of State, Gerhard Konow, helped to plan and encourage the efforts of the universities. As a result, this German federal state now has Europe's largest and most wide-ranging cluster of institutes for Japanese studies, at the universities of Duisburg (Japanese economics, social science and geography), Bochum (history, language and literature), Düsseldorf (gender studies), Cologne (traditional culture), Bonn (social science, history, language and translation), and Hagen (law), and at the North Rhine-Westphalian Institute of Language Training in Bochum.

At national level, the spirit of 1968 soon evaporated. When Chancellor Kohl visited Japan in 1993, for the first time since he entered office in 1982, the *Japan Times* wrote in a biting editorial, "Bonn's discovery of Asia comes 15 years too late". Also worthy of note is what the leading daily newspaper *Asahi* identified as Foreign Minister Genscher's "Eurocentrist foreign policy ... that has not taken Japan as a diplomatic partner ... and has further contributed to the estrangement between Tokyo and Bonn". It is because of this situation that Ronald Dore cites Germany in particular when characterizing the European–Japanese dialogue as a "dialogue with interpreter" (by which he means the USA).

These Japanese comments capture well a certain underlying attitude on the German side, particularly as regards foreign policy – but apply equally to Japan, which, like Germany, acknowledges the USA as its main global partner and only then attends to important relations in its own backyard. Yet the allegations do not quite hold true. The German government has indeed recognized the importance of communication with Japan (if a little late) and in particular has begun to promote cooperation in the field of science. The main impetus came from the then Federal Ministry of Research and Technology under Minister Heinz Riesenhuber.

As early as 1982, the Deutsche Morgenländische Gesellschaft called for a new institute to research the great traditions of East-Asian cultures (those of China, Japan and Korea). Its proposed location was Kyoto. After long years of consultation in the Science Council and at the Max Planck Society, it became clear that the terms of reference must be changed. The institute should focus on contemporary Japanese studies, though not to the exclusion of all but economics-based disciplines as voices from German industry had demanded. In 1988, Riesenhuber brought before Cabinet a proposal to set up a foundation named after Siebold and to run the German Institute for Japanese Studies in Tokyo. That institute began work in the autumn of 1988 and, in only a few years, has grown to 14 Fellows besides its Director, plus two librarians and five other employees. It has three fields of interdisciplinary study – the society, economy and culture of contemporary Japan – in addition to research into the history of Japanese–German contacts. Doctoral grants are awarded in all these areas. Thus there is now a research institute in Tokyo that goes far beyond the earlier Cultural Institute in terms of both staff and objectives and, crucially, is sponsored entirely by Germany. The choice of topics reflects German interests, a fact that has proved valuable and attractive for the Japanese scientific community as well, as it enables the institute to cover issues that are not immediately apparent to Japan and to make contributions to the debate that are likewise new there. A year earlier, in 1987, the Japanese–German Center had been founded as the successor to the Japan Institute in Berlin. It is sponsored by both countries and serves more as a meeting place and venue for discussion, conducting no research of its own. Its influence is nonetheless very wide.

There is never a lack of research topics for the German Institute for Japanese Studies or of debating material for the Japanese–German Center in Berlin. It was evident from the start that Europe, and particularly Germany, simultaneously faced the same, or similar, problems as Japan. The most pressing must be the phenomenon of the aging population. This is progressing far more rapidly and in a shorter time span in Japan than in Europe. Accordingly, whereas European or German experience was useful to Japan in the early stages, the situation has now reversed, and Japan must now find a solution that we may learn from. A related problem is that of medical care in old age. This is not an issue for the medical community alone. Technical progress and funding are equally important. But it does entail fundamental ethical considerations – whether based on the Christian world view or the Buddhist-Shinto religious tradition. The question of the moment of death, that is, the problem of defining death (brain versus cardiac), is as hotly debated in Japan as it is in Germany. Laws both on this and on organ transplants were passed by the two countries' parliaments at about the same time. It is unsurprising that there are deep reservations about these matters in today's Japan, still dominated as it is by a religiosity and world view that possess strong animistic elements. This brings to mind how, after the world's second ever heart transplant was performed at Sapporo teaching hospital, the chief surgeon became embroiled in great difficulties. such that no further operation of the kind has since been performed in Japan until quite recently (March 1999). Instead, there arose a sort of "transplant tourism" to the USA and Australia, which in turn has become one of the many causes of the familiar "Japan-bashing".

Likewise common to the two countries is the radical change in family structures, attendant on modernization, industrialization and centralization of the population, in favor of the nuclear family. With it, the problem of caring for older family members has become acute. It is associated with questions about the place of women in society, economic issues such as pension insurance, and the debate surrounding the introduction of insurance for long-term nursing care.

The collapse of the bubble economy in the early 1990s bestowed on Japan such hitherto unknown problems as unemployment – especially youth unemployment – and the shift of production to low-wage countries. Again, the problems are very alike. Germans speak of the debate surrounding "Germany's industrial base", the Japanese of "hollowing-out". While the crash in South-East Asia naturally hit Japan's industry head-on, and harder than Europe's, the threat of crisis in Russia and its effects on Germany provide a similarly arresting spectacle for Japan.

Safeguarding the environment has long been high on the agenda in both Japan and Germany, even if Japan does lack a political party dedicated to arguing the case as vocally as Germany's "Greens". Finally, long-overdue structural reforms (electoral, fiscal and governmental) have abetted popular disaffection with politics in both Germany and Japan, though national-to-nationalistic right-wing parties and youth movements are more a German concern. Nonetheless, changes in people's value systems are equally marked in Japan and, surprisingly, research by the German Institute for Japanese Studies reveals striking parallels with Germany.

Similar issues in foreign policy include assessing events of the Second World War, gaining a voice on the UN Security Council, participating in UN peace-keeping missions, deploying armed forces in crisis zones, and development aid.

Besides academic inquiry into such important issues by the German Institute for Japanese Studies and their discussion at conferences and symposia of the Japanese–German Center in Berlin, two bilateral forums have been set up to extend the scope of German–Japanese cooperation. During Chancellor Kohl's visit to Japan in 1993, he and Prime Minister Miyazawa agreed to call into existence a German–Japanese "dialogue forum" (comparable to Japanese-French and Japanese–British forums that had already been in place for some time). One year later, Kohl proposed the establishment of a German–Japanese Cooperation Council for High-Tech and Environmental Technology, to be chaired jointly by Professor Heinz Riesenhuber and Professor Mori Wataru (then President of the Science Council of Japan). Both panels meet annually to discuss bilateral issues.

The dialogue forum has already born fruit in the form of an agreement to set up a youth exchange program between the two countries, signed by Chancellor Kohl and Prime Minister Hashimoto on the occasion of the G7 summit in Denver. Themes for joint projects currently being discussed by German and Japanese scientists with representatives of industry on the Cooperation Council include telemedicine, clean coal technologies, transport problems in megalopolitan areas, and photovoltaics (with the construction of German-Japanese plants in Vietnam). The report of a conference on recycling building materials has already been published in German and Japanese. The Cooperation Council also promotes exchange programs, an example being the Young Leaders Exchange.

Another product of this cooperation is the appearance in 1998 of a book describing opportunities for German firms, *Japan ist offen – Chancen für deutsche Unternehmen*, by Heinz Risenhuber and Josef Kreiner. Japan is by far the largest market in Asia, particularly for German industry. And yet, though there is a large cluster of Japanese corporate outposts in Düsseldorf (and another of Japanese banks in Frankfurt am Main), there is minimal direct investment between the two countries, commercial joint ventures are quite rare, and the Japanese prefer Ireland, Britain and Belgium as production locations. The volume of German exports to Japan (with 60% automobiles!) is relatively low. At the same time, Japan's gross national product totals some $4.5 trillion a year, which amounts to more than 70% of the economic output of East and South-East Asia. Some 60% of the Japanese gross national product is spent on private consumption, still constituting a vast potential economic power that shows no significant sign of dwindling despite the current stagnation.

As the Federation of German Industries and its President, Hans-Olaf Henkel, never tire of pointing out, the "closed market" myth that discourages many firms from venturing into Japan on a larger scale is wholly unfounded and ought to be laid to rest in the interests of all concerned.

Besides the economic data given earlier, we should also note Japan's huge capacity for innovation, not only in (production) technology, but also in management and marketing. Numerous reports from experience bear witness to it. In the words of Ferry Porsche – to name but one example – the Porsche company would have been beyond salvation had it not adopted the world-leading production technology of the Japanese automobile industry (in this case Toyota's) in the early 1980s. Yet we also encounter here a guarded attitude that is in fact no more than a rehash of the Eurocentric prejudice voiced time and again since the Enlightenment period: that the Japanese are not "inventive". As noted earlier, this European stereotype of Japan has even been adopted as a self-stereotype by some Japanese. In the mid-1990s, a government commission chaired by Michio Okamoto, a doctor of medicine and the former President of Kyoto University, set itself the task of offering Japanese schoolchildren instruction on "more innovative thinking" in the classroom. Here, Japan completely overlooked the fact that the doubtless real problems of its schools (such as truancy and playground violence) are by no means limited to Japan and cannot be attributed to some peculiarity of the Japanese character.

This brings us to another crucial topic: that of education and Euro-Japanese cooperation in education, training and research.

We have already touched upon the various youth exchange programs of a bilateral nature (and specifically those involving Germany). A series of conferences held in 1997 and 1998 dealt with the problems of this field in detail: the Conference on EU-Japan Cooperation in Education, Science and Technology at the University of the United Nations, Tokyo, in autumn 1997, "Universities Building Bridges: New Forms of Cooperation between Japan and North Rhine-Westphalia" at Bonn in June 1998, and "Asian Values as a Cultural, Economic and Political Challenge for Europe: Current Avenues of Research and Means of Focusing Humanities Research on Asia" at Bonn in July 1998. The demands raised at these conferences by both sides, Japanese and European/German, and at all levels, regional, national or EU, are practically identical – and often match the findings of the reports already cited, published some 30 years ago, of Lord Scarbrough and the Hayter Sub-Commission.

But first I shall attempt to present the progress of cooperation so far in the specific case of Germany and Japan. General opinions on the current state of academic youth exchange programs, exchanges of post-doctoral academics, joint research projects, etc., diverge widely. Some (like one DAAD representative at the Tokyo office) describe it as "better than ever before", while others (including the Alexander von Humboldt Foundation) fear a "rapid dwindling of reciprocal interest". Accordingly, an objective assessment requires some numerical data from recent years.

The latest available summary data on student mobility are for 1993/94 (BMBF, "Basic and Structural Data", 1997/98), when 59,460 Japanese studied abroad, compared with 41,704 Germans. Mobility as a proportion of total population is thus roughly the same in the two countries, and somewhat greater in Germany as a proportion of student numbers. Of the Japanese, the great majority went to the USA (43,770 or 73.6%), all other destination countries remaining far behind (3.4% to the UK, and 1235 or 2% to Germany). German students, on the other hand, chose a larger number of destination countries (16.9% UK, 15.6% USA and 14.3% France), though far fewer Germans (161, or 0.38%) went to Japan than Japanese came to Germany. The picture is the same for other EU countries (the UK with 136 and France 116 supplying even fewer than Germany).

DAAD, the German Academic Exchange Service, gives more precise (and more recent) figures in its 1997 Annual Report, though the data are limited to students it sponsors. On these figures, 123 German undergraduates, 280 graduates and 41 young post-doctoral academics went to Japan on a 1-year grant in 1996. The figures for the Japanese side were 100 undergraduates, 195 graduates and 26 post-doctoral academics. Germans visiting Japan thus predominate in this group, though they are more than offset by the large numbers of Japanese students who come to Germany either at their own cost or on exchanges (1602 in 1995 and 1236 in 1993/94, see above). Despite the stated DAAD policy that Japan should remain the focus of its funding programs in Asia, Japan is far behind both as a country of origin and as a destination in comparison with the numbers exchanged with other

EU countries, and even with Russia: more than 1000 Germans went on DAAD funding to the UK and a similar number to France, whence 700 and 400 students respectively came to Germany; the figures for Russia were 538 and 1800, and for Poland 371 and 1523. The USA is the primary destination for German students, with 2568, while 810 Americans received DAAD grants.

This imbalance becomes somewhat problematic when the subjects studied are taken into account, though detailed figures are hard to come by in this regard. While it will come as no surprise that the Japanese are led by students of German language and literature, these are outnumbered by musicians. France bemoans a similar imbalance among grant-assisted students from Japan, most of whom aspire there to attend academies of art. Here, again, old stereotypes come into play. DAAD explicitly states that Japanese students of the natural sciences, engineering, law and medicine show a stronger bias towards America.

The exchanges with Germany also continue to suffer the effects of a recent change in the Japanese university system (as do exchanges with all European countries save Britain): on the advice of Keidanren, the Japanese business federation, the initial two-year course of general studies at university has been discontinued in favor of vocational training from the first undergraduate year onwards. The obligation to take a second foreign language was dropped at the same time. Formerly, students took English as their first foreign language and, in order of preference, German, French or Chinese as their second. As not even a tiny percentage of students may be expected to take German (or French) as their first foreign language, the number of grant applications for foreign study in Germany (or any other non-English-speaking country) will probably fall even further. In the absence of attractive career prospects as German tutors or professors on general studies courses, the numbers of German language and literature students in Japan will probably likewise fall. This will also impinge on the DAAD tutors program.

Various remedies are now being discussed: German universities might attract students of subjects other than German language and literature by teaching such subjects in English. Japanese universities, which were sooner to identify the “language barrier” as a problem, are working on similar offerings. A second option – one that can only be implemented by the Japanese academic community – would be to move away from German language and literature studies, with their still strictly philological focus, and towards German studies, either as an area study or as an integral part of a broad, social sciences-based course in European studies. Help can and must be forthcoming from Germany and Europe. It may even be possible to provide an incentive in Europe, in the form of Japanese studies with a contemporary focus. Europe's recent upheavals – German unification, the fall of the Eastern Bloc, the fall of the USSR, and the emergence of new states with the attendant dangers of ethnic conflict in the Baltic, in south-east Europe and in the Balkans – have made Japan aware of the need for European studies. After 1989/90, Japanese foundations (such as the Toyota Foundation) suddenly faced large numbers of grant applications in this direction from sociologists, social scientists, anthropologists and the like. Students of law, on the other hand, were primarily interested in issues surrounding German unity, EU integration and the adoption of the Euro – always with an eye to greater Japanese involvement with and within the Association of South-East Asian Nations (ASEAN), the Asia Pacific Economic Council (APEC), the Asia Europe Meeting (ASEM), etc., and to the adoption of the yen as a regional currency.

A further prerequisite for the promotion of study abroad is course comparability and mutual recognition of course and examination performance. Japan has adopted a system of credit points, an area where German universities still lag behind. Currently, however, only 30 of the 134 points needed for a degree in Japan may be gained abroad. The Ministry for Education is negotiating with universities to relax this restriction.

Finally, it would be highly worthwhile to link the UMAP (University Mobility in Asia and the Pacific) system enabling student exchanges between Japan, Thailand and Australia with the European ERASMUS/SOCRATES program. Mutual recognition of course performance by peer faculties would encourage students to study in other participating countries. The incentive will be all the greater when faculty and university cooperation reaches the level of staff exchanges and joint research projects. The new DAAD program introduced in 1998 to promote student exchange between German and Japanese partner universities is to be warmly welcomed in this regard.

There are now two new DAAD grant programs. The first is one that the Japan International Science and Technology Center

(JISTEC), a foundation of the Science and Technology Agency, has offered since 1988. In 1997, for example, it awarded grants to a total of 2090 natural scientists, enabling them to research and study at 140 research institutes, for the most part in Japanese industry. While the total number of months of study and research so funded for researchers from the USA has increased only slightly since 1989 (from 329.5 to 447.3 in 1996), the figures for Europe have risen continuously from 683 to 1813. A similar increase is observable for Germany (from 89 in 1989 to 234 in 1996), though the percentage share of the total for Europe has remained unchanged (13.3% in 1989 and 13% in 1996).

Language and Practice, a program run by DAAD itself, is now in its 15th year and awarded 39 places in 1996. It will gain in importance.

A program inaugurated by Prime Minister Takeshita in 1987, Japanese Exchange of Teachers (JET), is of negligible significance to non-English-speaking countries, there being little demand for, say, German teachers at universities, and even less at Japanese high schools.

Let us turn to academic exchange. Here, we have figures for Germany from the Alexander von Humboldt Foundation (1997 Annual Report). In the "eternal list of Humboldtians", that is, of all academics funded between 1953 and 1997, Japan appears second with 1814 (11.6%), just after the USA with 1821 and far ahead of India with 1103. In 1997, however, the proportions were different: then, Japan took only fifth place with 93 grant-assisted researchers (6.0%), after China (177), USA (155), Russia (131) and India (124). In 1998, these were China (164), India (133), Russia (129), and the USA (126). The Japanese share of new awards for 1997 is lower again, at 27 (5.2%) out of a total of 519. The position is similar with regard to Humboldt laureates: the 13 (out of 291) that came from Japan in 1997 again put it in fifth place after the USA (161!), Russia, Israel and Canada.

The greatest cause for concern, however, is on the applications side. There has been a marked fall in applications from Japan in recent years (from 71 in 1996 to only 45 in 1997, a drop of over 30%). Even more alarming is an observed reduction in the caliber of Japanese applications. This suggests, firstly, that Germany has lost its attraction as a science base and, secondly, that the bias towards America identified by DAAD holds true for the entire Japanese scientific community. Expressed in figures, the success rate for applications from Japan was only 3.4% in 1997, putting it in sixth place after USA, Russia, France, China, Australia, and barely ahead of Italy and Poland. Year on year, the number of approved Japanese projects fell from 38 in 1995 to 37 in 1996 and a mere 16 in 1997.

In one regard, however, the data from the Humboldt Foundation are very positive compared with the DAAD figures: the distribution of funded researchers and laureates across the various disciplines. Of the 93 Humboldtians in 1997, 60 were natural scientists (22 medical scientists, 12 physicists and 11 bioscientists), 26 social scientists (10 in German language and literature), and seven engineering scientists.

Since 1978, the Foundation has awarded the Philipp Franz von Siebold Prize to Japanese academics who have rendered a special service to mutual understanding between the two countries. The prize is awarded alternately to representatives of the social sciences and the humanities, again ensuring balance.

In 1978, the Humboldt Foundation began (under the Feodor Lynen Program) to fund German scientists wishing to study and conduct research abroad. In the case of Japan, it does this in cooperation with the Japan Society for the Promotion of Science (JSPS), a public-sector foundation under the Ministry for Education, Science, Art and Sports. Since the program began, Japan has always come second after the USA in terms of both applications and awards (in 1997 there were 47 applications from Japan and 25 awards – in each case 14.2% of the total). This program, too, covers an impressively wide range of disciplines.

Since 1997, the German Research Association (Deutsche Forschungsgemeinschaft) has awarded Eugen and Ilse Seidel Prizes each year to one Japanese and one German academic for furthering the cause of mutual understanding. While the first of these were bestowed on two highly regarded and deserving academics, the Association missed the opportunity to honor active new recruits who had not yet entered the network operated by DAAD and the Humboldt Foundation.

Regrettably, these last two German prizes have no equivalent in Japan. The prestigious Japan Foundation bestows an Annual Award and Special Prize, yet it was not until 1987 that an Austrian working in Germany (the writer of this article) received the Special Prize, and another two years were to pass before Alexander Slawik, the doyen of Japanese studies in Austria, was presented with the Annual Award. And it was not until 1994 that a German was finally honored, in the person of Heinrich Pfeiffer of the Humboldt Foundation. Roger Goepper, former Director of the Museum of East-Asian Art in Cologne, followed in 1997. Over the same period, awards and prizes were bestowed upon 16 American, seven British and four French academics. This reflects the traditionally inward-looking and, as mentioned earlier, until recently mostly philological nature of Japanese studies in Germany – and also the scant notice paid in Japan or elsewhere to German research findings, for the simple reason that they have almost always appeared in German.

A proposal to award a prize for the best Japan-related doctoral thesis of the past year to a German (or German-speaking) university and to hold a small symposium on the subject of the thesis – preferably in Bonn after its transformation from a seat of government to a European science center – has disappointingly not yet come to fruition. However, in 1999, the Society for the Promotion of Japanese–German Cultural Relations, Cologne (JaDe), established, again on the German side, a prize for the best scientific contribution to Japanese studies by a young scholar.

We should accord due recognition at this juncture to the funding granted under the various programs of the Japan Foundation. In the Japan Cultural Institute in Cologne, we are lucky to have one of the few European establishments (the others being in Paris and Rome) belonging to a foundation of similar rank to our Goethe Institute. Japan-related academic projects, research grants and guest professorships are well funded in Germany compared with the rest of Europe – though here, too, Europe still lags far behind the USA. Thus, while the Japan Foundation has established the highly influential Abe Foundation for Global Partnership exclusively for the USA and dedicated an Asia Center to its home region, the sole project conceived specifically for Europe is the Special Program for Japan-Europe Cultural Exchange, and that did not come into being until 1993.

To conclude this necessarily somewhat detailed survey of the current state of academic cooperation between Europe/Germany and Japan, we see that both have strong ties with the USA and that these ties are likely to strengthen further. The status of English as a lingua franca and Japan's deepening integration into a politically and economically already powerful Asia-Pacific region nurture academic cooperation between it and English-speaking countries such as Australia (where, already, more than 10,000 children learn Japanese at elementary school). The links between Japan and the nations of Europe (with the possible exception of Britain) are comparably weak and are set to become even weaker. Some reasons for this we have already discussed. The primary cause, however, can only be assumed to be mutual neglect – not to use a stronger word – in the political arena. Japan itself is partly to blame. For a long time, the "European disease" (or English or German disease) has been a source of amusement, with Europe regarded as one big open-air museum. It is still presented as such to the Japanese public, be it at home in the "exotic" *Oranda mura* (Dutch Village) in Nagasaki, the Spanish Village in Ise, or the "Glücks-Königreich" (sic) on Hokkaido, or on package tours to "do" Germany by way of the *Märchenstrasse* or *Romantische Strasse*. The beginnings of EU integration, on the other hand, have stirred up old fears in Japan, and Europe has suddenly become the root of all evil. When the European internal market began to take shape in the early 1990s, headlines alluding to the Star Wars films proclaimed "The Empire Strikes Back".

While Europe – despite scant initial knowledge – is now slowly beginning to heed Japan, Japan still lacks the resolve to form a more concrete and accurate picture of Europe. To cite a few examples, President Chirac, acquainted with East-Asian art history from his student days, has visited Japan more than 20 times. He and Tony Blair vigorously supported exhibitions by their countries lasting an entire year in Japan, with great success. Japan, in return, has exhibited its own culture in London and Paris, has set up a grand new cultural institute in Paris, and has founded a training center for European teachers of Japanese in London (which both Baden-Württemberg and North Rhine-Westphalia worked in vain to procure for themselves). Japan is also due to stage a Japan Festival in Germany in 1999/2000; however, the plans for it are embroiled in difficulties, and work has barely begun on preparing a German Year in Japan.

Academic research institutes maintained by each country in the other can be important sources of ideas and advice for politics and industry: the Maison Franco-Japonais and the German Institute for Japanese Studies ought to (and indeed must) provide informed opinion on current issues, in addition and with recourse to their basic research. The German Institute has already started doing this, for example with its studies on value change, the role of the state in the economy, and the problems of the aging population. Further such national institutes in Japan would be useful, but most useful of all would be an EU institute as is now being considered by Brussels.

In exchange, it is high time that Japan founded a European institute in Europe. As early as 1992, the private Waseda University saw this need and founded a Europe Center to observe the progress of European integration from Bonn. The state University of Tokyo and the private Keio University regrettably failed in their cooperative attempt to create an inter-university research center in Germany resembling the "centers of excellence" found elsewhere in Japan. The recommendation of the Conference on EU–Japan Cooperation in 1997, reiterated in 1998 as an invitation to Japan by the state of North Rhine-Westphalia, "to establish a Japanese Institute for European studies in Europe", was summarily dismissed on both occasions, with allusions to the current scarcity of funding and the absence of a legal foundation. Clearly, Europe must do more to promote the cause.

European research institutions in Japan and their Japanese counterparts in Europe cannot hope to succeed without the necessary language skills. Here, Europe lags considerably behind the USA. Knowledge of Japanese is only just beginning to extend beyond the domain of Japanese language, literature and area studies. At present, it is still the economics-based disciplines that tend to require it the most. So far, however, there are practically no plans in Europe to hold language courses in Japan for students of all disciplines, as the joint US–Canadian Inter-University Center for Japanese Language Studies has done with great success in Yokohama since 1963, the Japan Center for Michigan Universities in Hikone since 1989, or the Associated Kyoto Program of 13 Us-American colleges in Kyoto since 1972. Only the University of Tübingen runs a small Center for Japanese Language in Kyoto (founded in 1993), while Bonn, together with North Rhine-Westphalia, is are beginning to make similar plans. Japan ought to be doing the same, for, as we have seen, European studies are likely to become important in Japan just when the requisite language skills start to dwindle. The requirement, in the Science and Technology Basic Plan adopted by Cabinet in July 1996, "to raise the total research and development budget to 17 trillion yen by fiscal year 2000" should secure the necessary funding. The grand aim of this plan is ”to encourage exchange beyond sectors, regions and nations”.

Japan’s ideas here bear a striking resemblance to the European recommendations “to cooperate in research”, “to conduct cooperative projects, especially create a global network” and “to pool personal and technological resources in order to mitigate the expense of research and development”. If both sides put only some of their declared intentions into practice, they stand to regain the mutual understanding that prevailed once before, at the time of Meister, Kaempfer and Siebold.

CHAPTER 15

The Siebold Palais in Würzburg, a Memorial and Visionary Place

A. Berglehner, W. Klein-Langner, A. Thiede

Philipp Franz von Siebold, born in Würzburg on 17 February 1796, was to become one of the great scientists of the nineteenth century. His medical, scientific and diplomatic skills made him famous both in Europe and Japan. He made Japan accessible for Europeans. While his life and work are still held in high esteem in Japan and even schoolchildren have heard of him, his memory has largely vanished in Europe, even in his hometown of Würzburg.

Several places in Würzburg still bear von Siebold's name, such as the Sieboldgymnasium, a grammar school thus named in 1961, a street, a town grove and, since 1882, a bronze bust by Christoph Roth. Franz von Siebold's turbulent life, his scientific work and his contribution to relations between Japan and Europe, however, were only accessible to a small minority of people interested in history.

This astonishing and somewhat embarrassing situation was finally rectified in October 1985, when a Japanese delegation from the twin town of Otsu visited Würzburg and the Siebold Gesellschaft e.V., Bayerisch-Japanische Vereinigung was founded. The aim of this society is to keep Siebold's memory alive and to carry on the tradition of cooperation between Germany and Japan.

Various events were organized during the years that followed to increase public interest in von Siebold, the great explorer of Japan, in keeping with the society's ambitious aims. A Japanese week was organized by the towns of Würzburg and Otsu in 1988; several exhibitions of Siebold's collections and research were held, including an exhibition in the municipal archives of Würzburg in 1989; and further events took place during the Bavarian horticultural show in 1990, at the fortress in 1992 and in Würzburg's baroque buildings. Work also continued on a modest scale, including German-Japanese meetings, visits from Japanese guests and visits to Japan by people from Würzburg.

Inspired by the inauguration of the Siebold Memorial Museum in Nagasaki in 1989, an idea began to take shape among the members and friends of the Siebold Gesellschaft; their most ambitious plan was to establish a museum in the hometown of Philipp Franz von Siebold.

This seemed at first to be a rather distant goal, but it suddenly came closer to being realized when the Japan Shipbuilding Foundation offered DM 1 million to help set up a museum. This was the first step towards realizing the goal. A suitable building was soon found: the villa of a former brewery director situated in a small park in the Frankfurter Straße. Built in 1887, it is classified as a historical monument and is at the disposal of the municipal authorities of Würzburg. With its restricted funds, the Siebold Gesellschaft reconstructed the villa, spending almost DM 3 million on adapting the site to turn it into a museum. This was only possible thanks to the generous contributions made by many German and Japanese public and private sponsors. The Siebold Palais (Fig. 1), containing a museum and a German-Japanese meeting place, was inaugurated on 3 July 1995 in a ceremony attended by numerous guests of honour from both countries. In addition to the items owned by the museum relating to the life and work of Philipp Franz von Siebold and to nineteenth-century Japanese culture, there is a permanent exhibition showing various loans from different museums, archives, libraries and public institutions, some of which belong to the Brandenstein-Zeppelin family, the explorer's direct descendants. Several changing and special exhibitions, such as a collection of items from von Siebold's second trip to Japan (1859–1862), are also on display.

The Siebold Palais is designed to be more than a place to house exhibitions, however. It is intended as a place where different cultures and their historical records and people living in different civilizations can meet. It is designed to stimulate discussion and to encourage contact between the cultures. In the basement, in addition to the two museum shops, visitors can relax in a tea house or a Sushi bar, and in the attic there is a library and two apartments for friends and scientists. Events such as concerts, speeches and symposiums are held in the exhibition rooms. The Siebold Gesellschaft and its museum have thus taken on the task of imparting knowledge and encouraging an interest in and

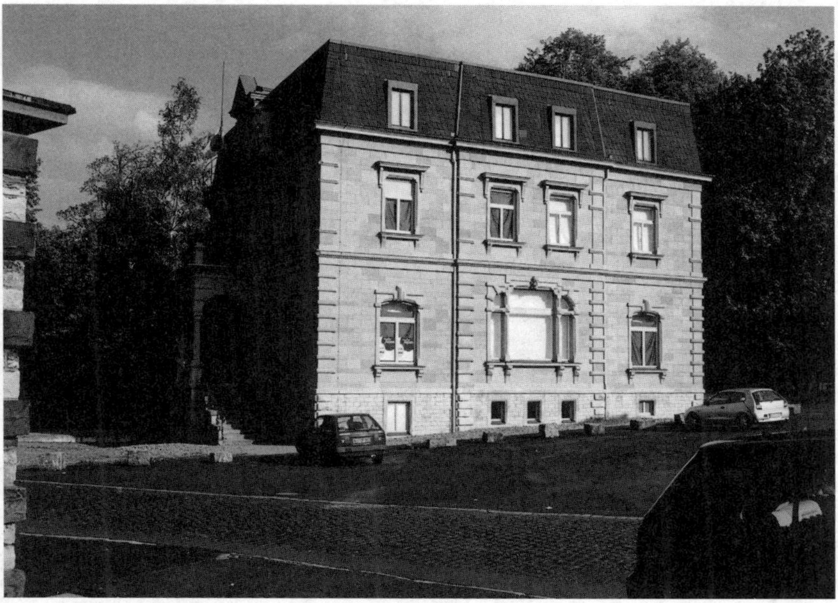

Fig. 1. The Siebold Palais in Würzburg

an understanding of each other's culture, making a modest but important contribution to the peaceful co-existence of different civilizations in accordance with von Siebold's work.

CHAPTER 16

Philipp Franz von Siebold and His Era – Future Perspectives:
Academic Cooperation and Exchange Between the Medical Faculties of the Universities of Würzburg and Leiden and Nagasaki University Medical School*

K. Wilms

In commemoration of the 200th anniversary of the birth of Philipp Franz von Siebold a Memorial International Medical Symposium with scientific contributions from the Universities of Nagasaki, Würzburg and Leiden took place in Nagasaki in September 1996, in order to acknowledge the merits of this outstanding physician and scientist and to initiate academic cooperation between the central sites of Siebolds' life and work.

The Past

Philipp Franz von Siebold was born in 1796 in Würzburg where the Siebold family had produced a dynasty of famous university professors with important influences in surgery, gynecology and obstetrics, internal medicine and zoology. At this time the Würzburg Medical Faculty was often referred to as the "Academia Sieboldiana". Siebold was educated in medicine and biology at the University of Würzburg. After graduating with honors in surgery, obstetrics and internal medicine he was appointed to the position of army surgeon in the service of the Dutch and left Würzburg in 1822.His skills were soon recognized by the Dutch authorities and he was appointed to the position of physician at the Dutch trading post at Nagasaki.

On 11 August 1823, Siebold arrived in Nagasaki and took over responsibility for the health management of the Dutch employees in Dejima, the artificial island which constituted the

* Presented for the Dean of Leiden, Professor Dr. P.J. Hoedemaker, and the Dean of Nagasaki, Professor Dr. S. Nagataki, by the Dean of Würzburg, Professor Dr. K. Wilms.

Dutch trading post and was the only connection between an isolated Japan under the Bakufu government and the western world in those days. Since the fame of Dr Siebold as a physician spread very rapidly, the Nagasaki magistrate soon gave him permission to treat patients outside Dejima. In addition, Japanese physicians were attracted from other parts of Japan and gathered in Nagasaki to be introduced to western medicine by Siebold. In 1824 he purchased a house in Narutaki, a suburb of Nagasaki, to teach western medicine to his Japanese students. In this way, Siebold not only created a school of western medicine but was also able to pursue various research projects in Japanese history and manufacturing, as well in the fauna and flora and geography of Japan.

In 1826, Siebold had the opportunity to travel to the capital Edo (modern-day Tokyo) for an informal interview with the shogun, which he used to make further observations of this – for the western world – so far unknown country.

In 1829, Siebold had to leave Dejima when maps and other items whose export from Japan was banned were discovered in his luggage. His Japanese collaborators were punished and he was forced to return to Europe. He went to Leiden where he received a warm welcome from the Dutch government. In Leiden he devoted himself to bringing the wealth of his information about Japan to the attention of the general public and the academic world. He published there his famous books, *Nippon*, *Flora Japonica* and *Fauna Japonica*, and established a museum to exhibit his collections. From 1859 to 1861 he was back in Japan. He once again gathered his former Japanese students in Nagasaki and by invitation from the Bakufu government gave lectures in Edo. He also treated Japanese patients and conducted research.

In 1863, Siebold retired from his position with the Dutch government and returned to Würzburg. He died in Munich in 1866, highly esteemed and honored by numerous European countries.

So Philipp Franz von Siebold, who lived and worked principally in three places – Würzburg, Nagasaki, Leiden – was the first physician to introduce modern western medicine to Japan. On the other hand he brought a wealth of information and invaluable scientific material from the as yet unknown country and rich culture of Nippon to the western world. As an interpreter of both cultures he exerted an enormous influence that has continued to the present.

The Present

In commemoration of Philipp Franz von Siebold, his 200th anniversary in 1996 was chosen – initiated and encouraged by the Dean of the University of Nagasaki Medical School, Professor Nagataki – to celebrate an International Medical Symposium in Nagasaki, together with the Medical Faculties of the Universities of Würzburg and Leiden, to lay the basis for scientific cooperation in the spirit of Siebold's heritage.

An Agreement on Academic Cooperation and Exchange had already been signed in 1989 between the Faculty of Medicine, Leiden University and the School of Medicine, Nagasaki University. A similar Agreement between the Faculty of Medicine, Julius-Maximilians-University of Würzburg, and the School of Medicine, Nagasaki University, was signed at the opening ceremony of the Siebold Memorial International Medical Symposium on 26 September 1996 in Nagasaki (Figs. 1–4).

The scientific program of the Symposium was arranged by the three medical faculties. The contributions on various comprehensive topics were presented by well-known scientists from the three faculties, thereby giving a good impression of the strengths and main foci of biomedical research in Nagasaki, Würzburg and Leiden. The topics of the symposium included radiation research, endocrinology, genetics, immunology, infectious diseases, defense systems, hematology, cardiology and otorhinolaryngology. From these presentations the audience could see that cooperation either already existed in different fields between the three faculties or could be established on the basis of close common interests.

The Future

At the closing session of the Siebold Memorial International Medical Symposium the three Deans – S. Nagataki (Nagasaki), P.J. Hoedemaker (Leiden), and K. Wilms (Würzburg) – stressed the intention of their faculties to implement the Agree-

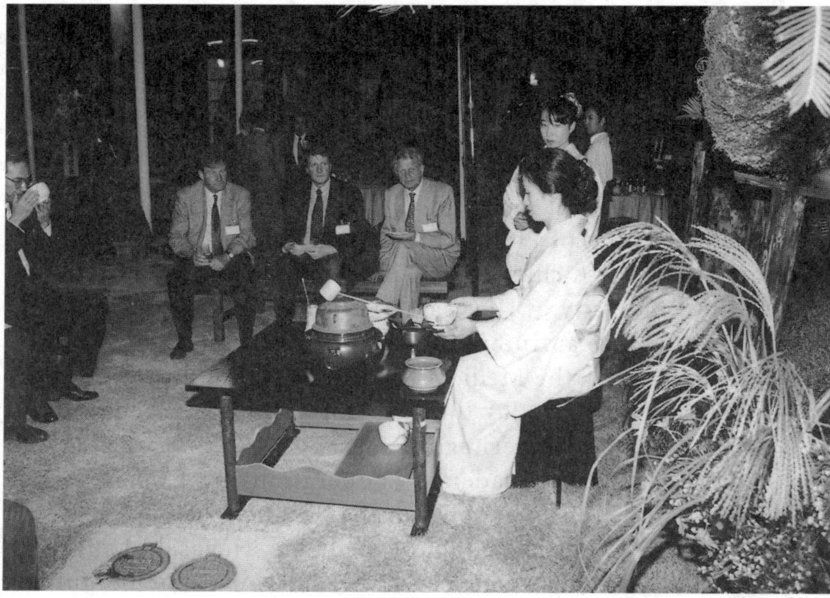

Fig. 1. Foundation event for academic cooperation, with Professor Thiede, Professor Hacker and Professor Kochsiek in 1996

Fig. 2. Professor Hoedemaker, Dean of the Medical Faculty of the University of Leiden

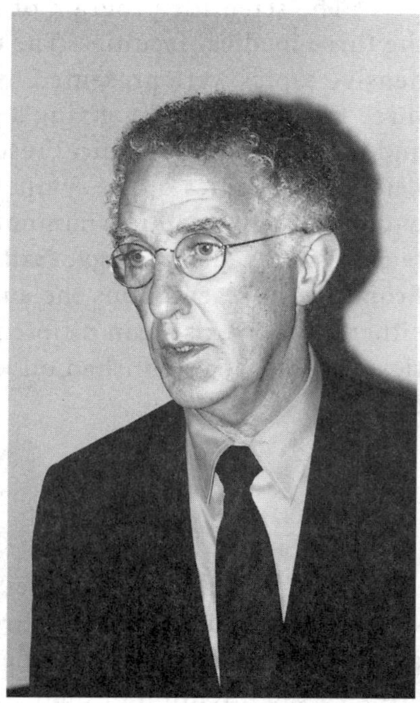

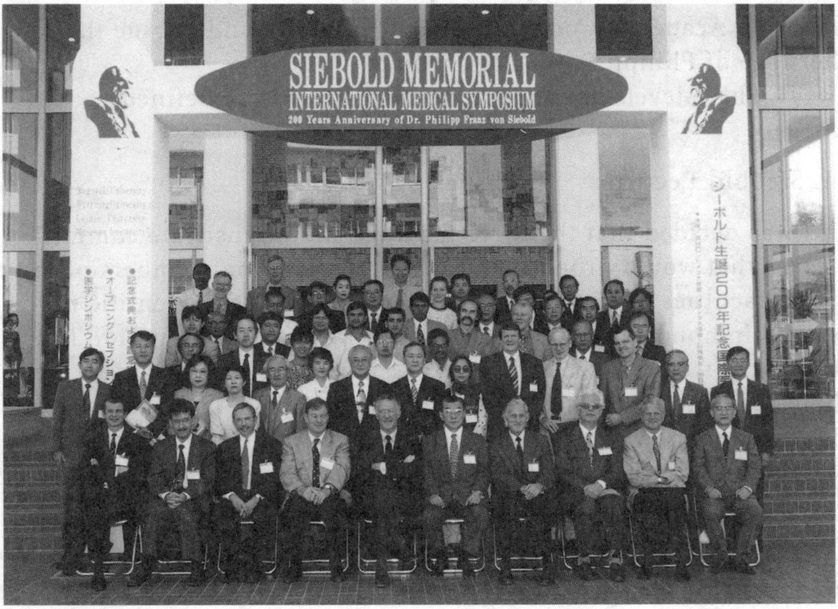

Fig. 3. Participants from Leiden, Nagasaki and Würzburg at the Siebold Memorial International Medical Symposium in 1996

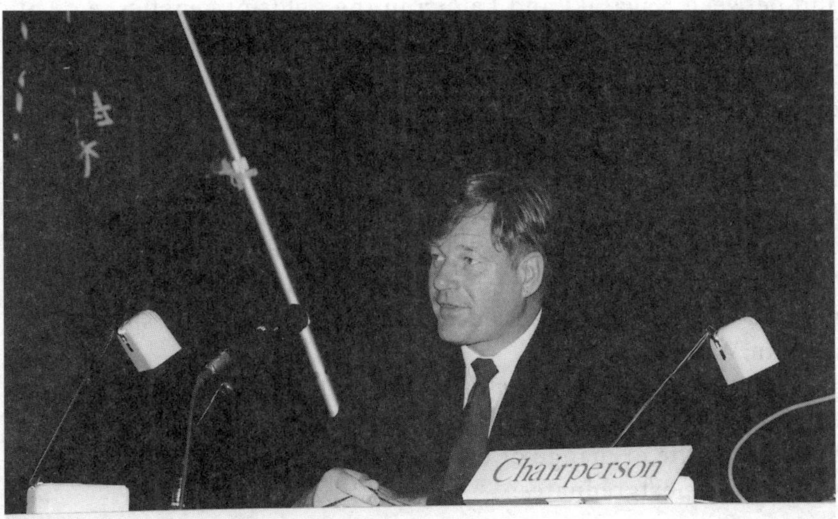

Fig. 4. Professor Thiede in the chair during the Siebold Memorial International Medical Symposium in 1996

ment on Academic Cooperation and Exchange and pursue the heritage of Philipp Franz von Siebold.

Three levels of cooperative modalities were defined:

1. Siebold Lectures

It was decided that the three faculties should institute committees that would propose and invite outstanding members of the other faculties to present Special Lectures on their scientific research in honor of Siebold and his work. The first invitation has been sent from Würzburg. In Nagasaki a fund for a Nagasaki Siebold Medical Award has been established. The Award's Special Lecture for the year 2000 will receive a prominent place in the ceremonies on the occasion of the 400th anniversary of commercial and cultural communication between Japan and Holland.

2. Scientific Cooperation

Lively and successful scientific cooperation had already been established before the 1996 Symposium between Nagasaki and Würzburg in the fields of radiation-induced thyroid cancer, in abdominal and transplantation surgery and in otorhinolaryngology, and between Nagasaki and Leiden in the fields of genetics, e.g., of neuromuscular diseases, and pediatric endocrinology.

From the contributions at the 1996 symposium, it was evident that cooperation in research in both experimental and clinical settings should be initiated in the fields of virology (HTLV-I and other retroviruses), bacteriology (molecular infections, *H. pylori*, respiratory infections), defense mechanisms (antioxidative defense systems) and hematology/hemopathology (adult T-cell leukemia/lymphoma, MALT lymphomas). Great attention was paid in Nagasaki to the advances in NMR imaging and spectroscopy in Würzburg.

It was accepted that closer cooperation in the above-mentioned fields should be promoted not only by sending material but also by the exchange of established scientists, postdoctoral fellows and postgraduates.

3. Education

The exchange of postgraduates and medical students of course raises the question of language barriers and the different government-regulated curricula. But the Japanese and European colleagues were all in agreement that the institution of exchanges at this level would be extremely important to a better understanding and closer cooperation.

The Nagasaki committee has now decided to send several fourth-year students to the Universities of Würzburg and Leiden for three months, to participate in the educational program including clinical exercises and research activities. A reciprocal exchange is to be pursued by the Würzburg and Leiden faculties.

For the individual students such an experience could be extremely important for their further development and future career. For the three faculties it is of the utmost importance to sow the seeds for a better mutual understanding and friendship between Europe and Japan in the next generation of academics.

CHAPTER 17

Closing Remarks

from:
"Proceedings, Siebold Memorial International Medical Symposium", Nagasaki, 1996

T. Ikeda

Distinguished guests, ladies and gentlemen:

It is a great honor for me to present the closing remarks at the Siebold Memorial International Medical Symposium. On behalf of the staff of the Nagasaki University School of Medicine, I would like to express my sincere thanks to all those who attended, especially from Würzburg and Leiden, and also to thank Professor Nagataki and the members of the organizing committee for arranging the wonderful scientific program.

We discussed many topics, including thyroid disease after the Chernobyl reactor accident, growth disorders, genetic diseases, cytokines, microvirology and active oxygens, hematologic malignancy, heart disease, and hearing difficulties.

I believe this medical symposium will lead to fruitful results and fond memories. In the course of this symposium, we learned that we have many research projects of common interest to our three universities. We also have ideas for many more research projects on which we can cooperate with each other. We had already concluded an agreement on scientific cooperation with the University of Leiden in 1989, and Nagasaki University and the University of Würzburg have now concluded a similar agreement.

For the 200th anniversary of the birth of Philipp Franz von Siebold, it was truly significant to have a symposium with scientists who are studying at the places where Siebold lived and worked. We are very pleased to have been able to hold the symposium at the historical site of Nagasaki in the memorial year, 1996.

We hope to be able to keep up our mutual communication and to maintain a long-lasting friendship. Thank you again for attending and participating.

CHAPTER 18

Remarks on the Future

from:
"Proceedings, Siebold Memorial International Medical Symposium", Nagasaki, 1996

S. NAGATAKI

As repeatedly mentioned, the aim of this symposium is academic cooperation and exchange between our universities, and the purpose of the scientific sessions is to seek detailed procedures for academic cooperation and exchange in the future, through scientific discussions.

On the last day of the symposium, the dean of each medical school summarized the proposals for cooperation from his own medical school, and the following table shows the proposals from the deans and from individual discussions between scientists from the participating medical schools.

I hope very much that this symposium is not only an event that commemorates Siebold but that it will also encourage scientists in our medical schools to undertake collaborative investigations in the future.

Production: Druckhaus Beltz, Hemsbach